The Key To Quantum Health

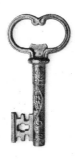

Awakening Your Highest Potential Through the
Power of Dynamic Nutrition & Empowered Thinking

By Shawn Stevenson

Copyright © 2010 by Shawn Stevenson. All rights reserved. No portion of this book, except for brief overview, may be reproduced, transmitted, or stored in a retrieval system in any form or by any means without the express written consent of the author.

Disclaimer: This book is sold for informational purposes only. Neither the author, publisher nor distributor of this information will be held liable for any use or misuse of the content herein. This book is not intended as medical advice and what you do must be the product of your own conclusions.

Cover Design by Kalin Gamble
Text Design by Camden Leeds, www.printnetinc.com
Text Layout & Design by Cindy Shaw, www.printnetinc.com

ISBN: 978-0-9845745-0-6

The Key to Quantum Health has saved the following resources by printing our book on 100% post consumer recycled paper, manufactured chlorine free, with bio-gas energy, and printed with vegetable based inks by **PrintNetinc.com**

24 trees preserved for the future	10,195 gal wastewater flow saved	1,128 lbs solid waste not generated	2,221 lbs net greenhouse gases prevented	17,000,000 BTUs energy not consumed

Review your reusing and recycling practices and invest in our future!

This is dedicated
to Carol "Mema" Stevenson.

You gave me everything,
and never asked for anything in return.
You showed me what unconditional love is,
and you believed in me so that I can believe in myself.
My life is in honor of you.

Acknowledgements

Mary Kariuki thank you for your conviction,
thank you for raising two beautiful daughters,
and thank you for allowing me to see my wife flower.

❦

Aunt Tikki, you are the one who inspired me
to write when I was just a little kid.
I love you so much. Thank you.

❦

My beautiful wife, Anne.
You are the most remarkable woman in the world…
Thank you for understanding me.
We are so fortunate
to be on this journey together.

❦

Mama Mukami, the world became a greater place
when you set foot on it. You created the space
for me to awaken, and that is the greatest gift to give.
Love and Gratitude Forever.

❦

Joann Cutis, you are more than an inspiration.
Just your presence gives hope to others.
Thank you for believing.

❦

Don and Lesa Brocksmith, a beautiful couple
who truly care about their family and their clients.
If you're looking for a home in the Midwest,
they will take the best care of you.

❦

Greg "Dagger" Whiteside. My good friend,
you are the protector of all,
I'm glad we found each other…
The world needs a strength
and heart like yours in it.

❦

Contents

Introduction 1

Section One
The Power of Right Thinking (Plus a little extra)

Chapter 1   Awakening 7
Chapter 2   Standing on the Shoulders of Giants 11
Chapter 3   Cracking the Energy Code 21
Chapter 4   Our Instinctive Desire 37
Chapter 5   Food, Appreciation, and Relationships 45
              Transcending Limitation 49
Chapter 6   The Ultimate Solution 57
Chapter 7   Discover Your Strength 65
              Make a Clear Decision 70
              Powerful Practice 73
              Asking the Right Questions 74
              Visualization Practice: Creation Station 76
              Where It All Comes From 77
              The Golden Ticket 79

Section Two
The Power of Right Nutrition

Chapter 8	Enzymes Reloaded	.83
Chapter 9	What Organic Really Means	.87
	What Do You Invest In?	.89
Chapter 10	Build Your Body with Intelligence	.93
Chapter 11	The Most Dangerous Ingredients in Your Groceries	.99
Chapter 12	Unlocking the Secrets of Water	.103
Chapter 13	Manifesting Physical Beauty	.109
	What Determines A Beauty Food	.111
	How to Get the Most Out of Your Beauty Foods	.113
	The Skinny on Fats	.114
Chapter 14	Welcome to the World of SUPERFOODS!	.117

Section Three
The Power of Bringing It All Together

Chapter 15	A Master Key	.133

Now It's Time to Eat!	.141
The New and Improved Kitchen Scenery	.142
Breakfast Note and SuperFood Drinks	.147
Extras	.159

	SuperTeas 161	
	Lunch Time 163	
	Power Salads 164	
	Entrees/Dinner/Supper 167	
	Life-Force Blended Soups 175	
	Dressings 181	
	80/20 Raw Options 186	
	Enzyme Inhibitors/Soaking Table 188	
	Fresh Juice Recipes 189	
	Good Food on the GO and Super Treats! 193	
Bonus #1	5 Essentials for Achieving Optimal Physical Fitness 199	
Bonus #2	Menu for Weight Loss 205	
	Additional Tips for Weight Loss 213	
Bonus #3	Menu for Increasing Muscle Mass 217	
	Additional Tips for Gaining Muscle Mass 225	
Bonus #4	Prosperity of Beauty Foods 227	
	Freedom to Succeed 232	
Resources	234	
About the Author 239		
www.TheShawnStevensonModel.com 240		
Index	242	

Introduction

What you will find within these pages is the absolute cutting-edge information for receiving, embodying, and maintaining levels of health and fitness that heretofore you may not have even known to be possible. I know that this is a valiant claim, but if the reader embodies just one of the teachings that are provided here in this book, it will bring brilliant change to your life that is simply unexplainable with mere words.

With the recent release of several films, books, and other multi-media pertaining to the fundamental laws of the Universe, it has become a very popular conversation among those that are "in-the-know" and wanting greater things for their life and for the life of the planet. What is revealed through studying these works, and then fully realized through personal introspection, is that you are participating in the unfoldment of your life's story at far deeper levels than you may have previously been aware of.

What quantum physics has unquestionably proven is that *everything in the Universe is made up of energy, everything carries a particular frequency, and everything is interconnected.*

What I have seen in my own experience, and what I have witnessed in working with countless individuals from all over the world, is that the most intimate factor in maintaining that high state of inspiration that you receive from reading a certain book or from attending a certain event, is directly determinant upon the *vibration* or the *energy* of the foods that you are putting into your body.

Most people are completely unaware that everything carries with it a particular vibration or frequency. You can easily go to a great event and be

Introduction

"uplifted," but if you turn around and put lower-level energies directly into your body, then it's going to bring your overall vibration down immediately. And which thing do you think is going to have a more direct impact on you? Is it the upliftment that you picked up from *outside of yourself,* or the low energy/low vibration foods that were just put *directly into your body?*

This is a powerful understanding, but it is a function of life that most individuals are totally unconscious of. To put it simply, it's just a popular practice that most people participate in. We'll go to a function and be uplifted and inspired, and then we'll head straight to the buffet or to a well-meaning family member's house and fill ourselves full of energy draining foods, resulting in an instant downgrade in the frequency we are carrying, and leaving us without the energy and the clarity that we truly want to have.

This practice becomes a vicious cycle that weakens us, and literally requires us to be dependent on the continuous stimulation and upliftment from outside of ourselves. Subsequently, this devolves to the use of harsh false stimulants just to make it through each day. And then we are left wondering *why* we just can't seem to make it over those humps. As a matter of fact, there just seem to be more and more humps constantly showing up! We simply are not living the life of abundance and passion that has become the popular conversation.

Prior to this, we just couldn't seem to make the real, permanent connections happen to receive the health, physical body, and life that we believe is possible for us. So the first key we need to understand is this: *Everything that you eat affects the way you think, affects the way you feel, and subsequently affects the vibration that you carry.* If you are someone who wants to truly step into your greatness, to maintain high levels of energy, as well as extraordinary levels of inspiration, then it is absolutely essential that you **fuel** your chosen path to success.

This is the "missing" component that I have observed in individual's lives, as well as in my own life, until I truly began to embody and teach the information that I have presented to you here in this book. When I did, and when other people do, it is as if the flood gates open, and all of the things that you read about, all of the things that seem to be so out of your reach, all of the things that seem to have been eluding you for so long, come rushing into your life in ways and quantities that are far beyond anything that you could have even imagined.

It is because of this critical understanding: You can read all of the books, you can attend all of the lectures, you can do all of the meditations, but if you are putting energies *directly into your body* that do not coincide or resonate with your ultimate goals, then you will always find yourself coming up short. This is simply because you are not *fueling* your path for success, for ultimate energy, for abundance, for self-realization. *You have to fuel your path towards your ultimate destiny.*

The reason that I put quotations above around the word "missing" is that these ideas and these incredible foods that I am presenting to the readers have not been missing at all. They have been here all along; it was simply that the public's awareness was not attuned to these things before. Instead of making a real, *powerful* choice, we have been making a *popular* choice. All the while, these amazing things have been waiting for the shift to take place and the people who are ready for unprecedented greatness to have access to them. This all comes full circle as an essential shift to understanding that you have to let *pleasure, right knowledge, and freedom* guide you all the way to living the greatest life possible.

What I have done in this book is unite the powers of *You Are What You Think About* and *You Are What You Eat*, marrying these two truths together to enable every reader to experience levels of phenomenal health, physical fitness, and abundance in all areas of life.

Introduction

These pages are loaded with specialized tools for transformation, details and knowledge about real Superfoods, and a plethora of recipes that will radically change your life and your body forever. Within these pages you will discover the truth about dieting, self-sabotaging behaviors, and how to quickly and easily receive *The Best Health Ever!*

All my best to you on your journey,

Enjoy!

SECTION

The Power of Right Thinking
(Plus a little extra)

CHAPTER 1

Awakening

What if you were holding in your hand the key to having the life, the health, and the body that you've always wanted to have? What if it were as simple as reading through a couple of pages to discover the *truth* when you've been disillusioned for so long about what is real?
Would you even be able to believe it?
Could it really be that simple?

Well, I'm here to tell you that it is that simple. And the good news is that we are going to do things the way that the entire Universe does things; with ease and grace. Most people have heard the saying, "If you try hard, then you die hard." And that's because it's not about working harder; it's about working smarter. It's about doing things a whole lot cleaner. Once you begin to understand the basic principles in this book, it will open up a whole new world to you that one might believe to be absolutely miraculous, but it's just the way that things really are, once you understand the *truth*.

In the context of working smarter, it's all about efficiency. It's about bringing immaculate quality and awareness to each individual act that you do. It is simply in realizing that for the vast majority of our lives we were doing the greater portion of the things that we were doing *unconsciously*. We had unknowingly created elaborate systems in our life for **not** achieving the results we wanted. This includes eating harmful foods, participating in detrimental behaviors and relationships, and not living the quality of life that is truly worthy of our highest self.

Indeed, some may argue that they were conscious and fully aware when they were eating the foods or participating in the activities that delivered them the state of health that they are now unhappily experiencing. But in truth, human beings are an entire species that is completely focused on steering clear of all identifiable *pain*. We will do most anything to avoid pain, or at least keep it to a bare minimum. Our lives are usually focused on putting things in order so that we don't have any trouble showing up later on.

Now, this being said, if an individual truly understood how a particular food or activity was actually damaging their health, and causing them to look and feel ways that they're dissatisfied with, then obviously they would consider trading it in for another choice. But the truth of the matter is that the vast majority of people in our society are completely unaware of what is really going on with the food that they're eating; what affects that food actually has on their body, mind, and consciousness; what it is that they truly need from the food that they're eating, and how to let pleasure, and not pain, be the guiding force in their life.

Pain is, indeed, a good teacher. But it is consciousness and pleasure that will ultimately guide you to having a life that is truly worthy of you. Like attracts like, and pain is an energy that resonates with (guess what) *more pain*. With higher intelligence developed, you want to use that pain as a discernment and get out of that vibration as quick as possible, as it doesn't have the vibrational energy to create long-lasting states of happiness and vitality. You will initially be happy to get out of pain; you will temporarily feel free, but it is just that, a *temporary* freedom. Your true state *is* freedom. You are free. Though at times, because of all of our societal conditioning, it doesn't always appear to be that way.

We want to move into an extemporal state, being prepared for all of the good that wants to come to us, while operating in the world with ease; no worry of time constraints and relaxing from the things that we "think" are working against us. This is activated by letting go of the lesser means of transformation, in place of higher and more insightful means; letting go of pain, and replacing that guiding force with a strong focus on pleasure. Not just temporary pleasure, but pleasure that is lasting and harmonious with everyone and everything around us; especially for our own consciousness, mind, and physical body.

Just because you may see somebody driving around in their car, talking on a cell phone and eating a sandwich, it doesn't mean that they're awake; it doesn't mean that they are fully alive and expressing to their life's highest potential. In the same regard, it doesn't mean that they're a lost cause either, or that they are less than you, or anyone else. It is most likely the case that they are simply not aware. Identification with harmful addictions can be fierce, but consciousness trumps everything. And it is not your duty to force change upon anyone else. That is a waste of good energy. All your energy should be directed fully, without hesitation, to becoming the best that you can possibly be. The greatest way to inspire change in others is by *being* the change yourself.

Now as we dive into the true essence of nutrition and right thinking in the next chapters, I present you with a couple of powerful quotes that resonate with some of the things that we have shared thus far.

> *"You cannot have anything that you're not willing to become in consciousness first."*
> —Dr. Michael Bernard Beckwith

> *"You must be the change you wish to see in the world."*
> —Mahatma Gandhi

CHAPTER 2

Standing on the Shoulders of Giants

On the surface level, the actual action steps in developing the body and health that you want are relatively simple: *Eat good food and exercise your body.* At first glance, you would imagine that this would be fairly easy for the greater portion of people to apply, but this is simply not the reality of the situation. If these two simple steps were all that it takes for people to experience the health that they want, why then are the vast majority of people continuously struggling with either one, or both parts of this equation? Why is it so rare that an individual actually achieves the state of health and beauty that they aspire to have?

If you look a little deeper you'll see that it's because the most vital piece in the whole process is not being fully addressed. The key to the ignition of the whole thing is not being used to turn the system all the way up, and instead the driver is constantly trying to push the machine to work.

From the perspective of real science, we would look and see that the results are not what we expected, so immediately we need to make a change in our approach. And in this case, the approach being a new and more intelligent focus on getting more leverage on the entire process.

The critical key that unlocks the physical actions of eating good food and exercising, and actually sets them on automatic for you, is putting your attention on shifting the *inner psychology* first.

Most people really do have good intentions when they start out. Their surface mind sets the intention to have a great exercise regimen, and live life with a new healthy diet, but their plans are usually doomed at the very onset. This is because their subconscious mind is *loaded* with all kinds of negative past conditionings, inaccurate assumptions about life, and self-sabotaging behaviors just waiting to pop up at any given moment and spoil the show. In essence, people are continuously attempting to go into their new lifestyle and achieve success, but they keep bringing their old-self right along with them.

All change is about becoming not you. You are becoming something greater than you define yourself to be right now. You are developing qualities and attributes that were not fully active within you before, and the critical point is that you need to do this consciously. If you don't develop yourself *consciously,* you may stumble upon some success, but the road will prove to be long and hard, simply because you didn't address the inner-game first, before taking action on the outer-game.

Rather than spending your time going around in circles trying to find out the keys to having perfect health, both physically and mentally, it is extremely important to recognize that the majority of society has been battling with the equation of diet and exercise for ages. What you want to do here is take a step back and look at the big picture, so that you can see clearly what's effective at getting results, as well as what's *not* effective.

The most intelligent strategy to take you where you want to be with the quickest, shortest, fastest route, and in fact, gaining massive leverage on your goals, is to address your inner-game first and develop the mind-set shifts necessary to lead you to your ultimate destination. One of the most critical mind-set shifts is *shifting the way you understand and relate to food.*

For the majority of our lives we were more-or-less blindly consuming food, and not really understanding the power and the value that this process holds. One of the most vital pieces of knowledge that you need to shift your awareness to is that ***food is not just food, it's information.***

The most intimate way that we interact with our environment is through the food that we eat. The molecular structures of the foods carry information that attach to receptor sites on our cells, which interacts with the information of our body. And this is happening *all the time*. Now by being aware and knowledgeable of this, we want to begin to consciously maximize the benefits of this process.

There have been many pioneers before us that have delivered critical information on what the most powerful forms of nutrition are, as well as the most energetic foods to give us the health and beauty that we desire. By learning from the individuals who have paved the way, you can turn decades of searching into mere days. You can take the direct information from the people who have discovered what actually works (right down to the distinct science and data to back it up), apply it to your own life, get the results, and then continue to build upon it for continued success.

Developing in yourself the underlying mind-set that food is information, when you look at food you begin to ask yourself questions like, "What kind of information does this food contain?" "What is this food going to tell my body to do once I eat it?" "Does this food have the information that I'm looking for to give me the body and health that I want?"

This leads to sharing one of the real life-changers that brings to light a huge piece in the equation of nutrition. It's not so much the basic insight that food simply carries different types of information; it's the understanding of whether or not the information in the food is even viable and usable in the first place. This brings to action the real mind, body, and energy connection.

In his landmark book, *Survival into the 21st Century,* Viktoras Kulvinskas gave scientific confirmation that *up to 85% of all of the nutritive value of food is lost in the cooking process.* This delivers a direct marker as to whether or not, the pure information that we want from our food is actually present and viable when we sit down to have a meal. This one discovery alone can straightaway give anyone enormous leverage to radically transform their health if they can understand this simple fact.

What made his work historic is that prior to the presence of his book, many people were utterly unaware of the damaging nature of cooking foods. There were many other great writers and teachers who put out phenomenal information on the subject that were also considered visionary, from Professor Arnold Ehret *(Mucusless Diet Healing System)* all the way to Dr. Norman Walker *(Vibrant Health).* But what Viktoras did was put together the cumulative proof. He compiled the data, he brought the facts together, and he presented them to the community in a way that had never been seen before. Included were the lifestyle aspects, consciousness aspects, and the scientific data. He recognized that there are many ways of being in the world and many different circumstances to live in. From this he presented tools for the achievement of right living and right nutrition in a growing paradigm of an industrial culture.

It was really no longer hearsay, or eccentric ideas at this point. Many of the great teachers of the past presented ideas that were profoundly true, but they were mostly based on their own personal experience. At most times throughout history, if you were going in a different direction than the popular culture, people wanted the facts, not what you found through your personal experience. Which is deeply ironic, because through personal experience is the only way that you can ever really know anything for certain. Everything else we hear about in our life is hearsay. If you don't experience it directly, then you cannot possibly know it to be true. *In order to truly know something, you've got to experience it firsthand.*

Remember this statement as you continue your process of discovery, and advancing through your successive levels of achievement.

This does not, by any means, limit things to the experiences of the common five senses, but in order for those dormant, untapped forces to be expressed within yourself, you must habitually and frequently cultivate the capacity of these vital forces. You must know what they are, your relationships to them, and put daily practice and attentiveness into nurturing them. This is what the Quantum Health phenomenon is all about. It is putting all of the pieces together in a divine flow, with a clear intention to reveal an outstanding human being.

We want to be experiencers of life, not watching things from the sidelines. We want to be participators in the unfoldment of our life's story, not have life disseminated to us by external circumstances. We are creators of circumstance, not victims of circumstance. Even if this understanding isn't within an individual's paradigm yet, Dr. Wayne Dyer put it beautifully when he stated, *"It is not your circumstances, but it is your attitude towards your circumstances that makes all the difference."*

Most people in our society are living vicariously through the people on television and in the media reports. This is how they are experiencing life; this is how they are experiencing the world. It is simply not authentic; it is the world presented to you through the eyes and/or the camera lens of someone else. And isn't it ironic how the word lens is actually a part of the physiology of our own eye and how we witness the world…?

Each individual must come to understand that you simply cannot take on someone else's view of the world and accept it as your own truth without experience and exploration into it. Your individual truth may be radically different from the next person's. And if you're not honoring your own truth, then you are creating a great amount of suffering in your life. You are forced to watch as your life becomes seemingly deficient because you have unconsciously acclimated yourself to someone else's definition of reality. You have accordingly adjusted yourself to seeing lack and confusion, while in reality you are literally surrounded by all of the amazing things that can create a life of endless enjoyment, if you only choose to live alignment with your own individual truth.

The trouble is that most people don't even know what kind of life they truly want to live. Again, they see the people on television and unconsciously view that as a marker for how good things are supposed to be. They think that what they are witnessing is the way that they should be in the world. And you can actually see the results of this ill-advised assumption everywhere in the actions and behaviors in society.

The answers that you really want to know can only be found in one place. Wouldn't it be utterly shocking that you were looking for an answer to a particular thing in every place except where the answer is actually located, and doing so because that's what everyone else is doing? (We'll breakdown the answer to this, and get into where the actual territory is at a little later in Chapter 7, "Discover Your Strength") In any case, if you want to know something for real, you must discover it for yourself. The truth is ever present and ready to reveal itself to you at any time. The most important thing for each individual to understand is *Truth is what works.*

A great example of this statement is even though hundreds, if not thousands, of people are being cured of so-called "incurable" diseases every day, rather than the popular culture asking and *understanding* how it is that these people are accomplishing such incredible feats, the public at large is still waiting around to get in the "big numbers" from some paradoxical, arcane establishment that has not brought forth a cure for much of anything, let alone providing people with right information to fully take control of their health and their life for good. The truth is that the people who are actually getting well are observably doing things that work. *Truth is what works.*

For years, Dr. Gabriel Cousens *(Conscious Eating)* has been helping people heal themselves of diabetic conditions and other debilitating diseases at his phenomenal facility in Patagonia, Arizona. This is a medical doctor with countless documented recoveries and factual clinical tests done. And time after time, diabetes is dissolved from the body, and health and vitality are restored within the individual. So why is it that the popular culture hasn't become aware of this yet? Dr. Cousens has successfully been providing his life-changing services at the Tree of Life Rejuvenation Center for nearly two decades, clinically tested and proven to work.

We also have the renowned Hippocrates Health Institute in West Palm Beach, Florida, headed up by Dr. Brian Clement *(Living Foods for Optimum Health)*. For over half a century, Hippocrates has been giving its phenomenal gift to society, enabling thousands upon thousands of people to rejuvenate their lives and completely heal themselves of their various diseases—from arthritis, to cancer, to diabetes. Hippocrates Health Institute has a full staff of health experts who focus on healing the whole person, not treating you like some type of machine and then sending you on your way. This establishment is focused on empowering the individual through right thinking and right nutrition, and providing the resources necessary for the individual to be conscious and successful throughout the course of their life. The results that they deliver speak for themselves.

These so-called "impossible" healings are happening and have been happening for years whether the unconscious public chooses to believe it or not; whether the people in control of the mainstream media choose to inform you of it or not. It is happening every day. Winston Churchill said, *"The truth is incontrovertible. Malice may attack it, ignorance may deride it, but in the end, there it is."*

The reality is that you have to be ready to hear the truth; you have to be ready and willing to step out of the "tribal consciousness" and into the awareness of ever-expanding good. If you don't believe it's possible, if you believe something is incurable, then you are bounded by that belief. And it is you and everyone around you who is forced to struggle because of this limited mental-setup. Until you let go of that illusory paradigm, and begin to focus steadfastly on infinite possibility, then this will inherently be your experience.

It takes just one idea to radically change your life and the life of the planet. Many of these ideas are now unfolding. It's not that Dr. Clement and Dr. Cousens' work is in vain and not changing the world. It has simply been a matter of the old "disease culture" paradigm fading away and becoming but a speck on the amazing story of the unfoldment of human potential.

The reason that their work has been so powerful and effective is their understanding that living foods have the right energetics to heal, rejuvenate, rebuild, and refine; allowing the individual's body to express its full potential. This is similar in scope to the work done by Viktoras Kulvinskas and the incomparable Anne Wigmore.

Mineral rich, fresh, living whole foods are the basis of optimal nutrition for the human body. Living food and living food advocation has been around since the beginning, simply because the information contained within these foods are of the highest integrity. It is our natural food source, and nothing has changed about that. It is just that our underlying conditioning of consumerism, and doing what's popular, has seen our health and connection to nature drop to dismal levels that have never been seen before throughout our history.

Many people, including myself, consider Viktoras to be the grandfather in the movement that has discovered the powerful energetics of living food nutrition. The implications and results have come to bear now in some of the healthiest and most brilliant people on the planet. When his work was released, action needed to be taken towards right nutrition, a reconnection to nature, and the activation of our higher potentials. His work was a significant breakthrough, and also a powerful catalyst.

Victor Hugo said, *"There is nothing more powerful than an idea whose time has come."* The Quantum Health evolution, the healing power of live foods, and a reconnection to nature is definitely an idea whose time has come. As a matter of fact, these things are now so powerful and enlivened that they truly cannot be stopped. So now we'll venture into the next chapter and reveal the source and substance of what's going on with the food that we eat, and how to unlock the vital energy that is resonating with unlimited power within each and every one of us.

CHAPTER 3

Cracking the Energy Code

To take everything further into understanding, not just "thinking," but to truly *understand* where we are actually getting our energy from, and what is so remarkable and transformative about living food nutrition, one of the first things that you need to realize with great clarity is this:

The average person uses upwards of 80% of their energy every day just to digest the food that they're eating.

This means that the energy you want to have to "get in shape", to work on your goals and aspirations, to do all of your day-to-day activities; if you're operating your body on the **S**tandard **A**merican **D**iet (SAD Diet), or a diet that is not conducive to creating vibrant health, then the vast majority of your energy is constantly being siphoned away to aid in digestion. And now your perceived energy capacity is rolling at a whopping 20% all the time.

This is one of the main reasons that people are not living the life that they truly want to live; they are tired, not feeling well, not enthusiastic about life, not out accomplishing the goals that they want to accomplish. There is literally an energy crisis going on, and it's not in some foreign land; it's in our own bodies.

Essentially, a large quantity of our energy is wasted haphazardly or unconsciously throughout our lifetime. And though this may be the common way of life for most of society, by gearing yourself up with the right information and empowering strategies, those common statistics, and that way of being in the world, can be shifted *instantly*, and abundant health and energy can move from the background to the foreground until it becomes your way of life.

Occasionally there are some people walking around "thinking" that they're feeling pretty good; they think that they feel okay, but they are really operating with just a fraction of the potential energy that they can be expressing. While most people already *know* that they don't feel good; they know that they're not feeling their best, and they are wanting desperately to have more energy to do all of the things they really want to do with their life.

We have an understanding that is seemingly encoded in the genetic makeup of each and every one of us. It is this deep feeling that *things can always be better, that there simply has to be* **more**. Of course, everything was okay before this; we made it out of our particular situations and circumstances; we "survived." But everyone knows that just "surviving" isn't the way that life was meant to be. Everyone feels that they have the potential for greater things residing within them.

What you can understand very quickly, if you *honestly* ask yourself if there can possibly be greater things in store for you; if there truly is a better way; if there are potentially greater things in store for your life, the answer will always be a deep and resounding *YES!*

Nevertheless, the reality of stepping out of the norm is so far out of the illusory paradigm of what's popular right now, that almost everyone seems to have forgotten about what it is, and what it takes, to go from just "getting by" to living a life that is truly worthy of themselves.

The key today can be chiseled down to *fueling your ultimate path.* In doing so you actually uncover the truth for what it is. You don't create it, you uncover it, because it is already here, and it always has been in its entirety. It is only your ability to recognize it, and to participate in applying it to master your life's potential.

It's simply a matter of knowing the *real* energy quotients. It's simply matter of applying one of the Universal Principles that is literally the *key* to unlocking unbounded energy for you.

You can enable yourself to have more energy and expand your consciousness *right now* to do all of the things that you want to do, and to begin living the life that you were truly meant to live. And it all begins with asking yourself a simple and powerful question.

That question is as follows:
What is the difference between having a vibrant, healthy body full of vitality and unbounded energy, or having a body that is tired, weak, and full of discomfort and disease?

Well, what I am providing you with is the answer to this question on the most fundamental level of understanding. Yet it is the key component in *all* of science and in *all* of health:

The difference between having a vibrant, over-flowing state of health or an impoverished, deficient state of health is the amount of LIFE-FORCE ENERGY that is flowing through your body at any given time.

Now you may ask: "What is this Life-Force Energy? And how does it 'flow' through my body? I thought it was all about dieting and eating health foods, and exercising like a maniac to get the body and life that I want to have. What is this guy talking about?"

To make a long story short, I have studied in-depth the physical, metaphysical, biological, chemical, and genetic workings and inter-workings of the human body, just to name a few. So the best method I feel to explain what Life-Force Energy is in this context would be metaphysically as well as biologically.

What's essential for you to understand is that the "Energy Field" or "Energy Being" that you are is actually measurable with hard-core science now. This can literally be seen or measured with several different modalities. One in particular is through *Kirlian Field Photography*.

For the sake of simplicity in understanding, Kirlian Field Photography is basically a system that enables you to photograph the "light" that you are expressing. You are able to see what the naked eye is unable to see, which is that you are, in fact, illuminated with Life-Force Energy. And the largest determining factor in how much light you express, or how much energy you are radiating with each moment, is dependent upon how much *bioelectricity* is residing within your cellular structures.

Bioelectricity is critical in the understanding of what vibrant health really is. Because your body is running on electromagnetic energy, it is the subtle energies; the phytonutrients, phytochemicals, and electrical energies of the foods you eat that truly determine the expression of sustained health and vitality. You are either increasing your "light" or bioelectrical potential with the foods you are eating, or you are decreasing it. You are either raising your body's radiant energy, or you are lowering it. Being radiant is an attractive force, and this is a tremendous insight to gain.

One of the main things that I've been asked almost daily working as a health professional is, "What can I do to have more energy?" Well, this is where true energy actually resides. You can try and trick your body by using false stimulants such as coffee, soda, processed sugar, and so-called "energy drinks", but understand that your body will inevitably look for its payback. These false stimulants put an enormous burden on your adrenal glands, which are responsible for regulating the stress responses in your body. This leaves you susceptible over the long haul to excess stress and anxiety, and increases the body's production of stress hormones like cortisol, which triggers your body to store more fat. On top of all of this, your adrenal glands are directly correlated with your kidneys, which can be considered to be your body's battery pack. Your kidneys are directly responsible for how much oxygen gets delivered to all of your body's tissues such as your muscles, your heart, and your brain.

So to feel good, *to feel really good,* your body needs oxygen, not a lifeless "energy drink." These popular habits literally destroy your kidney function (which is your real battery pack), tax your adrenals, and create addictions faster than you can say false advertising. This is why you see that if people don't have their coffee in the morning, or throughout the day, they just don't feel like themselves. It's really a deep struggle for them, and they feel as though they just can't make it through the day without it.

Most individuals in our society have a body that is extremely acidic. There are substances called alkaloids that are found in things like coffee and cigarettes that give people a temporary feeling of presence because those strong alkaloids seem to briefly neutralize the acidic condition in the body. But the prolonged use destroys the functioning of many of the major organs and vital processes of the body. The acidic condition is actually exacerbated as it reintegrates itself through the strong desire for more acidic foods. This is indeed an addiction and a vicious circle to get into. It is an attachment that leaves a person dependent upon a destructive habit just to make it through the day. This is not true living, or real freedom. This cycle can efficiently be overcome with the right tools and information; specifically, through awareness and the implementation of living, highly alkalizing foods (see Chapter 14).

The best news of the day is that with the profound understandings that science has gained about the real nature and function of the human body, and where we are actually at with technology right now, we are effectively able work along *with* someone's "vices". So if you are into coffee and coffee drinks for example, we can just add the most powerful Superfoods in the world right into that drink that taste absolutely amazing, and deliver your body massive nutrition right along with your daily coffee. So literally we can up-level your metabolism, deliver your body massive amounts of sustainable energy, and super-charge your immune system. All the while you get to have your daily coffee ritual that you've always enjoyed *while* experiencing incredible results that just keep building on each other and getting better!

The powerful understanding to gain here to bring everything full circle as a potent cognitive awareness is that the foods with the strongest electroluminescence (which can be seen with Kirlian Photography) are the foods that have the most aliveness or real energy potential. *Kirlian photography clearly shows that live foods have a tremendously stronger auric field than cooked foods.* Live foods are the only foods that can actually restore the microelectrical potential of the cells and thus the tissues. So you can ascertain that by eating live foods you are able to restore the real life-force and vital energy within your body. This is particularly excellent information to apply and practice. Especially since we are constantly exposed to weaker strains of food items and beverages, the introduction of the most powerful life-force foods (or Superfoods) provide your body with optimal nutrition to keep everything in significant balance.

The Brightest Light

We now enter into another key part of the overall Life-Force Energy lexicon that needs to become a deep-rooted understanding for everyone in our society. It's about the presence of the smallest physical units of light, which are known as *biophotons*.

The discovery of biophotons was one of the most historic and profound events in human history. Biophotons are stored sun energy that integrates itself into your cells in the form of tiny particles of light through the *living nutrition* you take in. You can absorb sun energy through your skin, as well as through the food that you eat. *Biophotons contain bio-information (life-information) that controls the vital processes of your body.* This is the master key in how we actually communicate physically with the entire biosphere and beyond.

What is most miraculous about the biophoton phenomena is that the creative source, or the energetic field that we are all a part of, is sending and receiving information from us 24 hours a day, 365 days a year, via the biophoton activity that is going on in and around our body and subtle bodies. This is such a powerful realization because those individuals who are feeling out of sorts or disconnected, and even the individuals who are wanting to deepen their connection to this creative source of energy, need to understand that it is literally through increasing the biophoton activity within your own body that your connection is automatically deepened. This is why so many who make the shift to living on live food experience a profound up-leveling in their consciousness, or what can be considered as having powerful spiritual insights and a reconnection to what is real and most important about who they truly are. Whereas before most individuals have only an esoteric idea of what spirituality is. Now they experience it for real.

Though the great spiritual traditions, teachers, avatars, and enlightened beings throughout our documented history have been speaking about our inherent interconnectedness and oneness with all of creation, it was Dr. Fritz-Albert Popp that formally discovered the presence of biophotons, and in doing so, showing that DNA (what contains all of the information about you) is an essential source of photon emissions (pure light energy).

He found that *97% of DNA was associated with biophoton activity,* while just 3% was filled with genetic information. This shows directly that light is continuously being absorbed and remitted by the cell's DNA and these biophotons have the utmost power to create, order, regulate, and express the individual's truest potential, which is naturally a state of vibrant health and well-being. These biophotons have the ability to raise the individual to higher and higher levels of being.

When you increase the light energy that is within your body, you are at a greater ability to make a *conscious* connection to the biophoton field, the creative source of all things, the Divine Source, or whatever you would like to call it. Everyone is connected to it, whether they realize it or not; whether they want to be or not; whether they understand it or not. There is truly *nothing* that is outside of it. You are having your entire experience within it, and this is where *all* of the information of each and every idea that has ever existed is located. Thoughts, ideas, situations, circumstances—these things don't just happen; there is a divine underlying order that is orchestrating it all. Your ability to up-level your wattage and consciously participate in this unfoldment is increased exponentially by bringing light energy into your body. Living foods are the only foods that express that concentrated light energy. It is truly a gift, and provided by the creative source with astonishing ease and grace.

The Key to Quantum Health

The Code is Officially Cracked

This leads us to the final piece in the trinity of what constitutes as Life-Force Energy, and this is where we are really going to focus our attention. The next factor is what can be considered the most vital part of our physical experience, so truly bring your full awareness to this.

What really puts you together, what really enables you to do all of the things that you do on a physical level, and what really holds the key to having the body, the health, and the life that you truly want to have are ***enzymes***.

Enzymes enable the body to do everything that it does on a cellular level, and in many ways on a metaphysical level. Without enzymes, you'd be just a pile of minerals and salts sitting there in your chair, essentially lifeless. Enzymes are catalysts that enable you to walk, talk, think, blink, digest your food, build your muscles, get in shape; and so on. *Enzymes are the chief component required to accomplish every function that your body performs.*

They are such a precious resource that your body has most of them locked away in the upwards of 100 trillion cells that you have in your body. This is a very efficient maintenance and protection system. It allows for you to live with high levels of energy everyday of your life, and to continuously experience vibrant health and beauty, as long as you are living in accordance with how your body actually works.

So, why isn't anyone really talking about this? I mean, you may hear about it briefly in science class, or you may hear about it randomly here or there, but most people have no idea that enzymes are the essential key to being *alive!*

People have been busy talking about counting carbs and calories, and only eating certain color foods (yes, there is a diet like that), and being on point systems, and laboring over never-ending cardio sessions and bizarre ab equipment that never seem to work. Now I don't know about you, but none of that stuff sounds pleasurable at all! As a matter of fact, I bet there are a whole lot of other things that you'd rather be doing than any of that stuff.

By taking a step back, you can clearly see that the whole system of commercialized health is completely irrelevant if you don't understand how your body actually works. By being empowered and learning about your body, you automatically begin to see an entirely different picture of your life. You start to see things become increasingly simple day after day, because you are finally developing the awareness of *what you're really made of, what you truly are, and what has actually been holding you back all this time.*

It is a powerful gift to be able to look at the past challenges and have the courage to recognize what doesn't work, and what has not served you justly in your growth and development. You can use that information as a discernment to know exactly what you *don't* want, so that you can move gracefully into what you *do* want, and to begin experiencing a life that is truly worthy of you.

Every individual should be an absolute expert on themselves. You literally live with yourself all the time! It is time to realize that, and to become conscious of what is most important about you, and how to unfold the health and physical beauty that has been within you all along.

In the understanding of the function of enzymes, you are intrinsically realizing what enables your physical form to take shape at the foundational level. *Enzymes only exist in living organisms.* They are basically like codes so that everything can do what everything needs to do. Whenever you eat a living food—an orange, for example—that orange has enzymes in it that assist in communicating to all of the vitamins, minerals, trace minerals, phytonutrients, etc., what they need to do once they're inside of your body. It assists your body in sending the goods where they need to go to do their job.

Here's the kicker and *the most important thing that you will ever hear on the subject of nutrition* (so understand this sentence, implant it in your mental rolodex, and recognize what it really means about you as you read further):

> ***All enzymes, biophoton activity, and bioelectricy are severely damaged—if not totally destroyed—when they are heated above 118°F!***

This means that when you cook your food above this temperature, you are destroying upwards of 100% of the *Life-Force Energy* that is in that food.

Now, unconsciously we might say, "Well, so what? That's okay. My body has enzymes in it, so when I eat that cooked food I'll be alright; my body will be able to do something with it. I'll be able to get by." And that's absolutely true, to some degree.

But what someone didn't seem to mention to everyone, and what has been forgotten in the equation is that *you have a **finite** amount of enzymes in your body*. This means that you will eventually run out of them, and when you use them up, then obviously your body no longer has what it needs to function and you will cease to exist.

Now I know that this may sound a little harsh at first; or something that you may not even want to hear, but when you understand this, and the impact that this has on your health and energy, it is truly *life transforming* because this is where you finally learn to take your power back. This is where you take control of your life and your health and begin to experience life the way that it is intended to be experienced; with vibrant health, unbounded energy, and with radiant inner and outer beauty that will inspire you and everyone else around you.

Understand with great clarity that *raw and living foods have enzymes in them so your body doesn't have to "waste" its own enzymes to break down a bunch of lifeless food that is put into it.* It doesn't matter if you are guzzling down a whole order of fries, a whole chicken, or a whole-wheat bagel; your body has to use its own enzyme stores to break that stuff down. Every time you put that lifeless food into your body, you are essentially withdrawing from your bank account and dying a little bit. That's why you feel tired in the afternoon after having a meal of cooked food. You are literally giving yourself a net loss every day. Because you are eating lifeless, denatured food, your body doesn't even recognize it as a "real food", so it also sets off an immediate immune system response. The end result for you is more sleepy time.

Your body could really care less about you getting in shape and expressing higher states of consciousness when it's trying to deal with a bunch of lifeless food that's been put into it. Humans are the only beings that cook their food, and coincidently we are also the only animals that get epidemics of cancers, diabetes, arthritis, asthma, auto-immune diseases, etc. Except, of course, for the animals that we feed. Our beloved family pets, who are eating the food that we give them, are also getting the same diseases that we get.

It's time to take the blinders off and see what's really going on here. Do you think that this is just a mere coincidence? You never see reindeer walking around with diabetes. You never hear about gorillas dying from some cancer epidemic. These things are so obvious that people literally can't accept it to be this simple. The truth is that most people think that they're making the decision of what they're feeding themselves and their family, when in fact the decision has already been made for them. There are basically 27 aisles of lifeless food to choose from at your local grocery store; a smoke; a drink, grab a video and a lottery ticket, and on your way out the door in hopes for a better life. This is the experience we have bought into for feeding our families, and this is what's continuously influencing the decision making in our lives.

The ironic part is that the majority of the 27 aisles of lifeless food are actually made from the same 10 to 12 foods! We have literally been missing out on over 99% of all of the other foods that are available in the world! So much variety, flavor, and abundance that can trigger levels of satisfaction in you that you never even knew existed. Yet we have been subjected to the bottom of the barrel, and trying to get by on what was unconsciously disseminated to us as a "square meal."

No way! Not anymore! Those are the days of old. Those days of hopeless hope are over. The truth is now being revealed with astonishing speed. Every day, more and more people are waking up and making *real, empowering decisions* to step into their greatness, and to take the best possible care of themselves and their families, because there is truly nothing more important than that.

The choices you make from here on out are going to tell the rest of your life's story. The food choices that you make express a great deal about the kind of person that you are, the kind of life that you are choosing to live, and how you are choosing to relate with the rest of the world.

At the most fundamental level of being, everything you eat affects the way that you think and it affects the way you feel. Becoming conscious of the basic raw materials that you make yourself out of is obviously of the utmost importance, because that translates up into the higher rungs of being in the world, and unfolding your ultimate potential. Without mastering this, going up into higher levels of being, such as the development of your intellect, working on your gifts and talents, expressing your creativity, the cultivation of your soul and spirit, will be tremendously difficult, if not impossible to achieve fully. All of these things are inherently going to be affected by how you feel because of what you are choosing to fuel your life on.

True, anyone can have moments of insight, or phenomenal creativity, but it's about consciously living in that state, being able to understand it, cultivate it, and access it at any time that you choose. You are indeed holding the key to the expression of your greatest potential.

At the most fundamental level, *real growth is about letting go.* This is what allows you to make room for new things to come into your life. For example, you can't have the healthy body that you want until you let go of the old, tired, weak one. You can't exclusively have the best food on the planet, that allows for you to feel good all the time, and experience pleasure every time that you eat, until you let go of the old destructive diet that has been holding you back all this time. You have to make room for the good to come in.

Until you do this, it will constantly be a struggle trying to fit things in that are literally resonating at two different frequencies. So what happens is they will continuously cancel each other out. You simply cannot walk around with two contradicting ideas about anything and expect to have powerful growth in your life. This is what creates the experience of always feeling like you're stuck in the same old thing.

It is as simple as letting go of the contradicting ideas, and taking complete responsibility of your mind. And with a clean slate, you now become more capable of thinking the thoughts that you want to think; harmonious thoughts that are fueled by a definiteness of purpose. Without definiteness of purpose, without knowing *exactly* what it is that you want and where it is that you are going, how in the world are you ever going to get there?

Now we are ready to take the next step in dissolving these illusory paradigms that are being recycled over and over again in our society, so that you are able to break free and make the decisions for living the life that *you* want to live.

It is *your* life, and no one else's. It is meant to be lived the way that you intend, but you need to actually have the courage to set your own intention. So now we'll move forward into bringing definiteness of purpose to the forefront.

We are literally entering into the next stage of our evolution. Are you ready? It is absolutely the best time ever to be alive. Let's continue on our journey because this is the start of something really, *really good.*

CHAPTER 4

Our Instinctive Desire

Every single person has an innate underlying desire to be *alive* and to experience vibrant levels of physical health. Every individual has an inherent need to experience the full spectrum of the abundances that life has to offer; from good health, wealth, and companionship; to continuous growth, integration, and self-realization. Most importantly, yet often overlooked, is the fact that every individual has an inherent desire to be conscious; to be fully aware of life itself, as well as the life that they are creating through the fundamental choices that they're making every day. This is the very reason why you woke up this morning. This is how at this very moment you are thinking, breathing, seeing, moving, feeling, and experiencing. Again with emphasis, *every single person has an instinctive desire to have excellent health and vitality.*

When a person does not have excellent health, they will intuitively feel that something is missing from their life. They will feel that something is wrong with them. If you are a person walking around with the idea that a part of you missing, then you will be in constant search of something to fill that void. This is where the *snowball effect* takes place; because if you are looking to the outside world to bring a sense of completeness to you, then you will always and only find a temporary solution. For example, you may unknowingly be turning to certain "comfort foods," or certain types of relationships, or maybe even a particular act or event to make you feel better about yourself, or at least allow you to lose yourself for awhile until your reality sets back in. Over time this behavior accumulates, resulting in unconscious addictions that have compiled so many hardships, problems, and excuses on top of you, that you don't even know where to begin to get your life back on track.

Understand very clearly that the first step in having the excellent health that you instinctively aspire towards is *taking 100% responsibility for your life!*

No more excuses, no more "he said this, or she said that." No more, "You don't know my story, and it's so hard." No more, "I can't" or "I'm not." Every one of these excuses creates your experience. Do you think that while you're complaining things are getting any better? Well, of course not. The truth is that as soon as you make a decision—a real decision—it immediately sets in motion a shift in the course of your life that will bring in a whole new set of circumstances, people, and resources that will change your life in the most amazing ways if you let it.

The trouble is that most people don't really know how to make a *real* decision anymore; one that can open up the doors for them, and really allow the good to come into their lives. The art of making a decision has been lost somewhere in the day-to-day shuffle that has lead people to experiencing life with this victim status, and struggling through life with a tremendous amount of fear and suffering. Life is not intended to be this way, and you know this innately. But if you never choose to take yourself out of that paradigm, and make a real empowered decision for your life, then you will obviously continue to experience life in much the same manner as you have thus far.

Now here is the apparent loophole or the proverbial "Pie in the Sky" theory that most people are walking around with: Almost everyone seems to think that they will be happy somewhere down the line in this magical place called *the future.* They say that all they need to do is just get to this certain point and then they will take the action that they have been putting off, and finally they'll be happy and at peace and enjoying the life that they've always wanted to have.

Everybody operating with this "somewhere over the rainbow" mind-set just needs to take a really good look at the results that this way of being in the world is yielding in their life right now. This is the exclusive indicator of whether or not that plan of action is working out for you. If you keep doing what you're doing, you're going to keep getting what you're getting. It is a very simple formula, as well as a profound truth. You have to stop living like a hamster on a wheel, and begin to bring some real confidence and passion into your life to experience what you want to experience *right now*.

The only time that really exists is *now*. This is all you have. How has seeing yourself as happy somewhere down the line after you get to such-and-such place worked out for you so far? There always seems to be something else coming up, because you are always living in *the future*. You know that having the life that you want is possible. If just one single person can do it, then that is proof positive that anyone can do it. You simply have to relearn how to make a real decision and take action today! This is *your* life!

The first step in manifestation is making a clear decision as to what it is that you truly want. You really need to be completely honest with yourself about it. There is nothing more important than identifying and knowing exactly where you are going because you are actually setting the course and destination that your life is going to be headed in. If you don't know exactly where you want to be, if you don't have a clear vision as to how you want your life to unfold, then you are likely going to end up just about anywhere.

When you have the power of a definite purpose and clear vision working within yourself, then you have tapped into a grand power that everybody wants to experience, and that is the rousing power of *passion*.

Passion lights the fire in you and keeps you focused on the manifestation of your particular vision. This is a force that the masses cannot stand against. Passion ignites the grand assistance of creative expression in you. So you wake up every day completely focused on what it is that you want to accomplish. It is an unexplainable energy in you that sustains your very existence, and allows you to do what some might believe to be the impossible.

I know it may sound relatively simple, to choose what you want, so that you can be passionate about it, so that you can live the life that you are here to live; but this is where the real crux of the situation resides. Most people don't actually know what they want, because they've never given themselves *permission* to want what they truly want. This may sound unusual, but it is the subconscious programming that's going on within the minds of the majority of people. It's simply a default setting we pick up from our social conditioning.

There is guilt, fear, and shame attached to wanting something greater for your life. It is a background message that plays in the manner of, "You can't do that." "You need to be more realistic." And most often it is in the form of, "Who do you think you are?"

That last quote from the mass collective voice is an incredibly empowering or disempowering statement depending upon how you look at it. One way:

"Who do you think you are?" is a blatant invitation to get back in your place; to get back in line and succumb to the status quo. That voice proclaims, *"You have no right to be great!"*

Even though there are a few people here or there that might tell you that you can do and be anything, that anything is possible for you, the resounding under-current of society is screaming at you to be "realistic," to be just another bystander. If you are not 100% confident in who and what you are, or at least in the real process of consciously uncovering that, you will undoubtedly be pulled back into the barrel and experiencing life much the same way as those around you. You will be living life on the default plan, seemingly disconnected from what is real and most significant about yourself.

Now let's take a look at the truly *empowering* sentiment hidden in those words: "Who do you **think** you are?" This very clearly reveals the truth about your ability to create your life based on the way that you think. *"As a man thinketh, so is he,"* as scripture would indicate (Proverbs 23:7). Your thoughts create your life experience. Your thoughts have actual physical substance, and quantum physics is quickly proving what has been known throughout countless civilizations, and taught by many of the great enlightened individuals, the reality that *your thoughts are literally the most powerful force in all of nature.* Your thoughts are the very substance that is creating the experiences you have every moment of your life.

When you awaken to this, when you understand this with all of your being, you have then discovered the essential nature and infinite power that has been residing within you all along.

So now, if you could do anything in this world, and you knew that you couldn't fail at it, what would it be? As a matter of fact, name five things, or ten things, or 100. Paint a picture of the life that you want to have. Not the idea of the life that someone else has for you. What is the life that you are meant to live?

This is what you are here for. The desire is there within you for a reason. If it is about your happiness; and especially if you are bringing joy to yourself and others, who are you *not* to be accomplishing these goals right now? You can literally write them down right here on the pages provided, or you can put them into your new journal of things that *you will* accomplish in your life. Then right next to each goal that you have for yourself, give it a meaning. Write down exactly *why* you want to have

Our Instinctive Desire

this in your life. Write down what it will mean to you when you accomplish this incredible feat. (This is tremendously important!) And as we continue our journey, you will be provided with master keys to manifesting the life that you are meant to live *right now*.

> *"The most important key to achieving great success is to decide upon your goal and launch, get started, take action, move.*
> —Brian Tracy

The Key to Quantum Health

Our Instinctive Desire

CHAPTER 5

Food, Appreciation, and Relationships

An essential step in achieving the life and health that you truly want to have is developing *a complete and intense appreciation for **yourself** and for the body that you have right now.*

Understand that when you have a *true* appreciation for your body, there are certain things that you simply will not do to your body. You will not put harmful food and other substances in your body. You will not neglect your body and deny it the freedom of movement and exercise. You will not disrespect your body through your actions and carelessness. It may sound strange, but when you truly appreciate your body, you develop a *closeness* to your body that will prevent you from even putting it in harm's way. When someone truly appreciates their body, they will give their body the very best possible nourishment. They will enable their body to flourish through motion and exercise. They will treat their body with the utmost *love* and *respect*.

Every single person wants to have a nice, fit, healthy body. This is 100% true because your body is the facility that contains your mind and your consciousness. Without a healthy body, rationality will tell you that the mind and the consciousness will not be able to express themselves fully, and the unfolding of your complete potential will be inhibited. *Your body is the facility through which you accomplish all things.* If your facility breaks down, then your whole operation breaks down. Your capacity breaks down, your output breaks down, your success breaks down, and your perceived value breaks down. In order to achieve true success, your body needs to be vibrant and have an infallible capacity to endure.

Food, Appreciation, and Relationships

So now I pose some questions to you:
How do you achieve true health?
How do you attain true physical fitness?
How do you achieve true success?

The answer to all of these questions can be summed up in five simple words:

YOU ARE WHAT YOU EAT

Now, everybody has heard this phrase before. But most people have never made it a clear understanding. *Every single thing* that you put into your body sets in motion a chain of events. Everything that you put in your body causes a shift in your cellular expression. The body that you have now is basically the result of what you have put in it over the past several days, months, and years.

Additionally, every single food and beverage is, in fact, a stimulant. Every single stimulant that you are exposed to has a direct and immediate effect on your mind and your physical body. And it's not just the food that you put in your mouth. You are also feeding yourself with the information that you take in—what you listen to on the radio, the people that you talk to, your circle of friends, what you watch on television, what you read, *what you think*. Science has proven that the information that you take in actually rewires, re-creates, and reconnects the synapses that form the physical network of your brain. To put it simply, the information that you take in actually becomes your flesh!

Knowing this, it is important that you now become more aware of the environments that you put yourself in, the information that you take in, and most importantly, *become more conscious about what you think!* We've all heard the adage "food for thought" when in fact it's more accurately depicted the other way around, "Thought for Food." What you think determines what you see. What you *think* determines your actual experience.

Let me give you an example. Let's say that an old vintage 1969 Mustang with a couple of dents and some chipped paint pulls up at a stop light where you and your friend are waiting to cross. Now, let's say that you have a great appreciation for cars, but your friend (quite the opposite) only knows about newer Mustangs that they have seen around town or on television. So your friend thinks that it's just some ratty old car in front of you. But you, on the other hand, see an incredible piece of car-making history; a car with potential. *You see beauty.* The car pulls away, and the two of you cross the street. You leave the situation feeling happy, feeling interested, feeling inspired. While your friend leaves the same situation feeling indifferent; and if anything a little bit annoyed.

Now can you see how your thoughts create the experience that you have? Two people can be at the exact same event, at the exact same time, and have two totally different experiences. As a matter of fact, a *thousand* different people can be at the exact same event, and have a *thousand* different experiences and points of reference. *No two people experience things the exact same way.* You and only you inhabit that body of yours. No one else feels what you feel, and no one else experiences what you experience. It is your body and yours alone. No one else sees through your eyes. You are the constant observer of your life. You and only you determine the way in which you will experience each moment. This holds true for every single moment that transpires in your life. You simply may not have been aware of it before.

You bring the emotion to each moment. It's not the other way around, nor has it ever been. Societal conditioning has taught us to let the external environment dictate how we feel all the time. Basically experienced as:

What's going on in the world = your state (or the way you feel)

When in reality it's:

Your state (or the way you feel) = what's going on in the world

Every thought that you think has a correlating chemical that is released into your body. For example, just the thought of sex literally changes your physical body, but most people have never examined this or questioned this *thought* instantly manifesting change in the physical world before, simply because it's such a common experience. Most everyone takes for granted how this actually works. Your thoughts affect your physiology *immediately,* and this is a fact. So understand this very clearly: *You literally get to choose how you feel all the time, and it will instantaneously create your experience.*

A great example of this is when you are in love with another person. The feelings and emotions that are flowing through your body are literally *all you*. The person that you are in love with didn't come by and sprinkle magical fairy dust on you to make you feel that way. They don't have some unrelenting power over you. It is something that you created within yourself, and it is there and available for you to have access to all the time. It is always your choice to express it or not; and it is literally your choice to live in this state all of the time, no matter what the conditions are around you. It is simply about the cultivation of this way of being by doing your inner work.

So for now, practice bringing the emotion that you want to feel to each moment. Practice bringing love to the moment. Practice bringing excitement to the moment. Practice bringing peace to the moment. Practice bringing happiness to the moment, and very soon you will begin to see that the joy that you were looking for "out there" was within you all along. That is what freedom truly is.

Transcending Limitation

Now as far as most "outer world" relationships go, the difference in perception among people is why there are so many self-proclaimed enemies, enemies by association, and erroneous critics in the world right now. Everyone is, of course, entitled to their own opinion. But when there is a lack of understanding of a particular point of view, we usually shun it, detest it, pass it off onto someone else, or ignore it all together. If only we would take a moment to understand it with an open heart, we would see clearly that at the root of all things there is goodness. *It is not just about tolerance; it is about true acceptance.*

When you begin to see the beauty in all things, when you begin to appreciate all things, your experience becomes one of unending enjoyment. You see, just by appreciating more things, you experience more pleasurable moments. Understand that if you live in this state habitually, your life becomes one incredible event after another. This may sound like a far cry from the popular definition of reality, but that is due only to limited thinking. If you remove the boundaries from your mind, you will see that we are, in fact, *unlimited* beings.

Merely a hundred years ago, we thought that we were limited to staying on the ground; the idea of flying was absurd! A few centuries before that, we thought that we were limited on how far we could travel on this planet, for fear that we might fall off the side of the Earth. (This was actually taught in universities!) Even more recently, about sixty years ago, in fact, we thought that we were bound by the confines of this planet. Now countless people are experienced in space travel. Understand very clearly that we place all of the limits on ourselves. We are the ones who don't think that we're good enough. We are the ones who think that we don't deserve this or that. We are the ones who are hindering our own progress by not taking full advantage of the unlimited potential that is constantly pulsating inside all of us. This capacity is always ready manifest, and demonstrate who we truly are!

Food, Appreciation, and Relationships

The complete unfolding of the human spirit is directly influenced by the facility that it is contained within. Being compelled to fulfill our potential, in all areas of life, is correlated directly to human nature. So if everyone has this same intrinsic need, why then are there so many who are disillusioned and failing at having the health and life that they truly want to have? Is it an accident? Is there some outside force that wants to see so many people sick, overweight, out of shape, unhealthy, and unhappy?

The answers to these questions have many sides. But first, for those who have faith in a higher power; understand that your Divine Source does not want to see you in a bad way; does not want to see you hurting; does not want to see you unhappy; does not want to see you depressed and unsuccessful. It simply doesn't make any sense. In basically all spiritualities, the very meaning of God is *Love*. True Love is *unconditional*. It only gives; it doesn't take away. Your Source has given you this life to be anything that you want to be, and to flourish. *Your Source has given you this life to **be** the good that you wish to see on this planet,* so that your light shines brighter, and so that you can be an inspiration to others. Dr. Wayne Dyer articulates it like this, "You come from a source of well-being, and you must be like you what you came from."

For those individuals who do not believe in a higher power, understand that you do still have tremendous faith. You have faith that you will wake up in the morning. You have faith that if you make any action, there will be a reaction. You believe that you are conscious and that you are alive. You believe this is inherently true because you are experiencing it *right now*. You have within you the capacity for so much.

If you are truly conscious, then you will understand that your choices create your life. If you want to flourish, you have to take responsibility for yourself, and do the actions necessary to be the success that you truly want to be.

*If the above is true in both cases, if we have an innate need to **understand** and to be **successful**; why then are so many people still failing at health and success?*

Though your thoughts and choices create your own experience, we all have collectively created this entire world as we know it to be. There is a simple answer to the question of why there is seemingly so much lack of success and shortfalls in the health of so many:

> Our recent history's *collective consciousness* has created this world based upon the dominating mind-set of lack, limitation, competition, and a sense of separation from each other, and most notably from ourselves.

If you look at a map of the entire world, you will see a bunch of lines that separate each country; that separate state from state; that separate these people from those people... But the funny thing about it is that those lines aren't really there; they don't even exist! *They are imaginary borders!* They're just drawn in. As a matter of fact, you weren't even around when they did the drawing. You were not there when it was decided that they were going to divvy up the land and say, "These people go over here...and these people go over there... Okay that's good... so now we have a country!"

Obviously we are "separate" now because those people are not in our country... And they have their own country anyways, with different lifestyles and practices that are different from ours... So we must be separate... *Right?*

Please understand, you weren't even there when they made the decision to do any of that stuff. You were just sort of born into it, and now you go parading around with a sense of separation and unconsciously limiting yourself, because as a result, you have built borders and boundaries in your mind.

When people are fighting and operating in fear that someone will take something away from them, or get something that they don't have, or that the resources might run out, or they might lose a prized possession, or they might miss out on an opportunity, or that there has to be a winner and a loser, there will inevitably be turmoil within their mind. And this limited mind-set will always lead to suffering.

When people are operating from a competitive mind-set, they will eventually do whatever they think they have to do "to get by," even if it's detrimental to the well-being of others. To put it very simply: It is no accident that so many people are sick, overweight, unhappy with themselves, and struggling constantly to have the success that they want to have. The conventional system is set up that way. It is set up for you to fail.

When you spend your money on the food that is making you sick, someone is getting paid for it. When you spend your money on the medication that you need, because of the food that's making you sick, someone's getting paid for it. There is an inconceivable amount of money to be made in the creation and maintenance of sick, out-of-shape, unhealthy people. Hospitals have to stay in business, right? The synthetic food companies have to stay in business. The drug companies have to stay in business. And where does all of the money go if you remain vibrant and healthy?

That's right…There is no money in those businesses if people remain vibrant and healthy! Are you starting to see how all of this comes together?

The competitive mind-set that created this farming of sick people naturally fears that people will wake up to this. The competitive mind-set feels that there is lack, so they create and advocate sickness to be certain that the money continues to flow into their pockets. But the competitive mind is greedy and it is continuously creating *more* sickness, just to try and abide the fear that they might lose out on the acquisition of more. So now sickness has been stretched to epidemic proportions. No one wants to say it, but you don't have to look hard at the environment around you to see that vibrant health is a far cry from the norm.

Though the way the system is set up is not an accident, it is still inside the individual to choose which path they are going to take. It is human instinct to make our choices based upon the information that we have. If you don't know of a better way, then how can you go a better way? Because we are unaware of our full potential, we generally do only what we know how to do from the world around us. We receive our habits from our parents and from our peers by default. We have even sunken to the point that we are actually taking health advice from people who aren't even healthy! We are taking advice on life from people who are not living the kind of life that they teach about. It simply doesn't make any logical sense!

If you are taking advice from anyone, in any field, who is not getting the results that you want to have, stop following them immediately! If you continue on their path, you will end up exactly were they are at right now. If you want a new and *better* way, you have to get on a *better* path! This is the intrinsic way that human evolution manifests itself. Someone steps outside the realm of conventional thinking and *creates* a better way. Against all odds, against all nay-sayers, and with the embodiment of real faith that they will succeed, individuals have created the ways of life and the luxuries that so many of us enjoy and even take for granted today.

It is through creation that everyone will flourish and reach their full potential. It is through creation that disease, pain, misery, and ill health will be a thing of the past. It is the creative spirit that will enable all people to prosper; whereas the competitive mind-set will inevitably fail with the increasing consciousness of those who have been debilitated by believing in it.

People are tired of being sick, they are tired of being out of shape; they are tired of seeing their friends and family suffering from *preventable* diseases. People are tired of not having the energy that they were designed to have, so that they can do the things that they want to do with their lives, and unfold the true potential that is waiting to be expressed from within themselves. *The People are ready for change.*

Now marks a critical turning point in human history. Those who become more conscious will thrive as never seen before throughout human evolution. Those who choose to remain unconscious will diminish under the control of the last remaining powers operating on the competitive field based on fear and greed.

You get to choose right now which path you are going to take. By reading this book, you are choosing to up-level your consciousness. You are choosing a path that is going to lead you directly to the health and success that is so closely linked to your very existence. It is an incredible path that will breathe new life into you. It is a path that will supply you with answers to the questions that have been eluding you for so long. You are being handed the keys to your new life. From here on out, you write the story of how you want your life to unfold.

Be clear in your mind that you acknowledge and embody the truth that is within you, appreciate all of the successes you achieve, and have an unimaginable amount of fun and enjoyment every single day!

"If we all worked on the assumption that what is accepted as true were really true, there would be little hope of advance."
—Orville Wright
Along with his brother, built & flew
the first recorded flight of a heavier than air craft

CHAPTER 6

The Ultimate Solution

If you really want to live the rest of your life with the body, the health and the energy that you want to have, then the first thing that you need to do is **_Throw out your ideas about "diet" right now!_**

All of the magazine articles and books you've read promising you the body you want, all of the tips that you've gotten from so-called health experts, all of the diets that have come and gone that promised to deliver you the secrets to finally getting the health and the body that you desire… But in the end, they all landed you right back where you started, and likely worse off than before. Throw all of that stuff out! The illusion is over starting now!

The overwhelming truth about diets is finally being discovered by the public. People are tired of being sick; they are tired of being out of-shape; they are tired of not feeling good about themselves; they are flat-out tired of being tired. Let's begin by revealing the actual truth about diets.

FACT:
Statistics show that approximately 98% OF ALL DIETS FAIL.

Now let's let that sink in for moment…
As a matter of fact, I'll repeat it again so that you can get a clear picture in your mind as to why poor health is as prevalent as it is right now.

FACT: APPROXIMATELY 98% OF ALL DIETS FAIL!

The Ultimate Solution

This is a profound truth that most people don't even know about! And do you think that 98% could possibly be an accident? It's not very likely. Most people are unaware of this shocking truth, and they are just waiting around for the next new diet to come around so that they can hop on that boat leading them right back to where they started, "screw-this-diet-ville." And there are literally *millions* of people on hopeless diets right now, even as you're reading this page. So take all of these ridiculous diets, throw them away. They simply don't work, and a 98% failure rate should give everyone just a little hint that there is some serious deception going on.

The very word *"diet"* has a very strong stigma attached to it. It is one that creates a feeling of *deprivation* and *restriction*. That very word signifies impending hard-times and struggle. Although many times diets are for a greater good, let's be completely honest: each diet has a definite ending point that people are anxious to get to so that they can *get back* the things that they had to *give up. This is why diets do not work!*

Diets are about taking away things that people actually enjoy, and replacing them with things of far less personal value. Diets truly are about deprivation and restriction. Feeling deprived and feeling restricted does not make us happy. If you're doing something that does not make you happy, or does not make you feel good, then it's bound to fail. Feeling deprived and feeling restricted cannot create true health...it is simply illogical. How can punishing yourself actually make you happy? How can avoiding what you really want, lead you to getting what you really want? It simply doesn't make any sense. The only occurrence that *does* make sense in this existence is getting from one reward to the next. This can be described ultimately as a transition.

Life is filled with transitions. It is deep-rooted in human nature to want to continuously transition to something greater. Once we have achieved something, no matter how big or how small—it could be within seconds, it could be within minutes, it could be within days, or it could even be within years—we will inevitably grow tired of it and seek out something more.

For example, you might achieve a higher level of physical fitness than you have right now, but then you'll want to become even more fit, not go backwards! You might have a degree; now you want to get a better degree. You might have a nice car; now you want to get a nicer car. You have a big house that you live in; now you want to get an even bigger house. You're making a nice amount of money; and now you want to make even more money. And so on and so forth. This is a continuous cycle that can be found at the root of all so-called "driving forces." The critical thing to understand here is that many times people fail to recognize all of their possible choices, or they fail to recognize that they even have a choice at all.

When you lose the understanding that you have the ability to *choose* to have everything and to *choose* to have nothing, this results in stagnation. When you lack the understanding that you do have a choice, you inevitably become bounded by that mind-set, which consequently becomes your reality. You are living life on the default plan. This is where people develop an overwhelming feeling of being stuck and living the same thing over and over again residually, just counting down the days until they can get a break. This is the exact reason why people love to take vacations so much. It is their opportunity to get away from their lives, which they truly can't master because they are too busy feeling trapped in it.

This overwhelming feeling results in a blockage of the transition of a person's "driving forces" into becoming their actual reality. The resulting

The Ultimate Solution

complacency causes a tremendous decrease in the energy that *drives* a person to be all that they can be. Without the connection between those driving forces, and feeling responsible for one's own life, a person can never truly feel fulfilled.

This limiting mind-set does not end until a clear understanding is achieved and a greater importance is developed. The realization needs to occur that a person can actually break free from their default lifestyle, and begin to live the life that they truly want to live; a life without boundaries and life without fear.

When you live in a state of stagnation, fear keeps you trapped in that dark place. It actually becomes comfortable. People tend to fear change and making new choices because it makes them feel uncomfortable. It gives the blocked mind comfort to know that things won't change. *It gives the blocked mind comfort to know that the responsibility is not their own.* You are, in essence, living a deception that you put yourself right smack in the middle of.

When a change in consciousness is achieved, it becomes incredibly liberating for a person when they grasp the realization that they are in complete control of *all* of the choices that they make, and thus they are in complete control of their own life. Every single thing that happens in this world is based directly on the choices that people make. Every single thing that you do in your life happens when, and only when, you *first* make the choice to do it. You can't even get up out of your chair until you first make the choice to do it. Your heart doesn't even beat unless your brain tells it to do so. Now, who is in control of your brain? Is there some ghost in the machine making everything happen? Science can't find it… So guess who the sole responsibility is left up to…that's right, *you.* You are living in a finite body and you are controlling every single thing that is happening with it at all times, either consciously or unconsciously, with the choices that you make.

Now truthfully, you really don't beat your own heart. Most people don't even know what their heart is made of, let alone how to operate it. Consciousness itself does that, and that is what you *really* are. But on a physical level, if something is manifesting with your body, either positive or negative, it is the direct result of the choices you've made. You can make choices to hinder the functioning of your heart and other organs of your body, or you can make choices to improve them. It is intrinsically connected to the choices that you make every moment, as well as the choices that you have allowed others to make for you. And understand very clearly: *Allowing is a choice you make also.*

You choose to go to your stressful job, you choose to eat the foods that you eat, you choose to be around the people that you're around; you choose to do every single thing that you do in your life. If you chose not to do all these things, and to do something new and different, then obviously there would be new and different results that you'd receive. But do you *have* to do any of these things? Of course not! You make the choice to do them, and subsequently, these choices create the "story" of your life.

It is tremendously empowering once you understand, *truly understand,* that you can have something *new,* simply by making a *new* choice. You can have something *better* simply by making a *better* choice. One might complain that they don't have any other choice. This is, again, common in limited thinking. It is simply the case of not *seeing* all of the possible choices because of the strong identification and mentality that there aren't any other choices that can be made. If one continues to make the same choices in their life, they will inevitably continue to get the same things that they've been getting. This is purely the bounds of logic and reason. Yet, beyond logic and reason exists something that delivers your choices to you in an unwavering manner, which is determinant only upon your ability to *receive* what it is that you have chosen for yourself.

When you understand that you are not alone in this world, and that your "little world" is not all that there is; that you are indeed part of a

The Ultimate Solution

broader picture that is greater than anything that your surface mind can even comprehend, then you will understand that the universe is actually working with you, and conspiring to assist you in having every experience that you choose to have.

If you continue feeling that the world is against you, then the entire world will continue to be your enemy. You will continue to be limited to what you can fight and claw for in a self-defeating battle of *me against the world.*

Success is simply a mind-set to embody. Choose to be successful in whatever endeavor you embark on, and you will inevitably be successful in it. While this may sound relatively too simple, the overwhelming reality is that most times people have a *little* hope of success placed on top of a *whole lot* of doubt and worry. If doubt and worry is your *real* underlying mind-set, then guess what you'll get more of…? And to take it a step even further, doubt and worry are two primary components of what we commonly referred to as S-T-R-E-S-S!

Stress is the real reason that people are not happy at their jobs; the reason they're not sleeping well at night; the reason they're habitually eating the wrong foods, and the real underlying reason why so many people are out of shape, unhappy, and are *still* looking forward to that vacation.

Once you allow stress to drop into your life and become your ultimate driving force, then unconsciously your life's mission becomes strongly focused on ridding yourself of it.

Guess what this means in the experience of your day-to-day life?

If you're constantly working with, towards, and against all of the stress in your life, then you've given that stress a strong purpose. You've given it dominion over your attention, so consequently you've already been defeated by it. This is because your predominant mind-set is **stress.**

Now that we've gotten this simple truth to the forefront of your awareness, it's time that we do something about it.

To activate some powerful momentum, we're going to use the laws of logic to begin to gain some leverage on shifting the focus of your mind.

Your life is directly dictated by the mind-set, or the predominant thought patterns that you are maintaining. This is a law of nature. No one else sees the world through your eyes, no one else experiences the exact same things that you experience…so no one can feel the way that you feel. No person, place, thing, or idea can control you unless you give them silent permission to. You are 100% in control of your life…all you have to do is act accordingly. *When you make the choice to stop letting the external environment dictate your internal environment, then you immediately become the beneficiary and no longer the victim.* When you fully understand this concept, and encase it with your heightened state of consciousness, it is then that you have truly mastered your life.

A change in your mental set-up is all that is required. There is actually a change happening in you right now as you're reading this page. There is a change happening in your body chemistry as your mind is processing and storing information. Something powerful is changing in you right at this very moment. All you have to do is let it happen. You've already made the decision to look into this further, to keep reading, to keep searching for more answers…for more possibilities…for more truths. It is an continuous search for answers that leads us to different points in our lives. It is an uncanny need that we are endowed with; the need to find out what we really want; the need to find some type of meaning. It is this quest that has continuously driven humanity throughout the ages. It is truly perplexing for the answers to have been hidden in such a place that almost no one would choose to look. It is beyond words and beyond

The Ultimate Solution

reason when you realize that all of the answers that you have been looking for, and all of the meaning that you have been hoping to find, has been, and always will be, found waiting patiently inside of *you*.

When you realize this, you will realize your inherent greatness. All you have to do is be still and quiet enough to listen. All you have to do is move your ego out of the way, and let it happen. Everything that you hear, everything that you see, and everything that you read about just provides you with directions. None of these things have the answers, and *all* of these things will lead you directly back to *you*. The choices that you make from this point forward are going to create the rest of your life. Is it going to be the life that you want, or the life that you don't want?

The decision resides where it has always resided… *within you.*

> *"You have that within you which is ever impelling you*
> *toward the upward and advancing way;*
> *and that impelling something is the divine Principle of Power;*
> *you must obey it without question."*
>
> —Wallace Wattles

> *"Twenty years from now you will be more disappointed by the things you didn't do than by the ones you did do. So throw off the bowlines. Sail away from the safe harbor. Catch the trade winds in your sails. Explore. Dream. Discover."*
>
> —Mark Twain

CHAPTER 7

Discover Your Strength

During the early part of the 20th century, quantum physics came to the forefront with landmark discoveries that completely shifted the face of science forever. This was a historic time that was layered by the works of great minds from Albert Einstein to Werner Heisenberg. The discovery that was at the height of it all, and what has dramatically changed the way in which we interact with our world today, is that the entire Universe, our world, and our bodies are made up of **99.999% ENERGY.**

Nobel Prize winning quantum physicist Max Planck, in a speech given in Florence, Italy, stated the following:

"As a man who has devoted his whole life to the most clear-headed science, to the study of matter, I can tell you as a result of my research about atoms this much: *There is no matter as such.* All matter originates and exists only by virtue of a force which brings the particle of an atom to vibration and holds this most minute solar system of the atom together. We must assume behind this force the existence of a conscious and intelligent mind. This mind is the matrix of all matter."

The Universe is literally a vibratory field. Everything in it is operating at a particular frequency; everything is carrying a certain vibration, including *you.* This is why you can pick up a cell phone, for example, and communicate with someone on the other side of the planet, and not even be in each other's physical presence. Your voice is literally being carried across this vibratory field and received by someone at the other end. How are you able to do that?!

Your voice, which is an unseen energy (or vibration), is transmitted over miles and miles through the unseen instantaneously, and showing up at a particular receptor site, regardless of circumstances, without strain or struggle, and without you consciously knowing how it works.

Most people have never put their attention on this, nor the remarkable application of this power that you are metaphorically swimming in, because it's just something that's a popular occurrence. Everyone has a cell phone now, but almost no one considers the *miraculousness* of the situation, and that your little box with the number pad on it, isn't what's allowing you to communicate with people all over the world whenever you "call" upon this power.

The frequency that you *are*—the vibratory field that we are all a part of—is inherently interconnected. For the purpose of this particular discussion, we will focus on this understanding that everything is connected, energy cannot be created or destroyed (there is only *one* energy), and everything has a certain vibration or frequency.

Life has a certain vibration. A young, vibrant fresh-picked fruit has a certain frequency that is bright, radiant, and intense in nature. Of course, this can now be seen through Kirlian Field photography. Death also has a certain frequency; and the energy of pain, suffering, torture, fear, anxiety, and sadness all carry a certain frequency. And if it is being expressed *anywhere,* you are inherently picking up on it. It is a quantum phenomenon known as *entanglement.*

So if there is harm being done to someone, or war, or animals being killed and eaten for the entertainment of the senses, we are all picking that up on some subtle level, and that's just the way it is. Just as you pick up the good vibes from your family pet when you are hugging them, loving them, and petting them, that energy is transmitted out into the field. These are sentient beings also, and if any of the animals (like the ones that many people choose to eat) are experiencing pain, fear, anxiety, or suffering, then that is transmitted into the field as well.

Just as you *feel* that communication with your family pet, it doesn't need to be said, you just know that it's there. And if you pay attention, you can feel this with any person or sentient being. You can feel and understand what they are experiencing. It's just that most people don't have the courage to look and see what is really going on. They are afraid to see the truth. Most people would rather remain in the dark than choose to come into the light, and take the necessary steps to put forth healing, the energy of respect, and noble right relations into action. The energy of Love, compassion, joy, forgiveness, and gratitude are all truly higher vibrational energies. They literally trump everything else. It is so powerful and so simple that the surface mind can't really wrap itself around this. It is completely experiential.

Due to social programming, we have been taught to sweep a lot of this under the table and to remain docile and mediocre. You don't even need quantum physics to tell you any of this stuff; you innately know it to be true. These teachings have been around since the beginning of documented human history. That we are all connected; That there is only one power; That Love conquers all; That your thoughts create your reality; That your life is exactly the way you believe it is, and if you change your beliefs, you change your life; That you are made up of the same stuff as the creative source, and you *must* be like what you come from.

We've been taught to remain safe and sheltered, and stay in the status quo. And look at where that illusory way of being has gotten everyone. It has inhibited most individuals from stepping into their greatness. The mental borders have basically ushered in the onset of the most destructive conditions that we have ever seen our society in. The United States is experiencing the highest rates of illness, the highest rates of crime, the highest rates of drug abuse, alcoholism, debt, depression, disease, and I can throw a whole bunch of other negative sounding terms in here, but for what? They all have to do with one thing. And that is being out of alignment with who and what we truly are.

All of these things, which have been transmutated into current situations and circumstances, are there to enable you to wake up and step into your greatness at any time that you choose, so that you can begin to live the life that you were meant to live. A life that is becoming of you, and honoring to your source that downloaded you here, because in truth, you didn't just create yourself. And it surely wasn't your parents!

Do you know how much genetic coding, and chromosome patterns, and double helixes, and amino acid profiles, and electromagnetic energy has to go into that tiny dot that is less than the size of a pin prick when you were created? No disrespect, but most parents don't even know how to work a remote control! Now, my life experiences may convey to individuals that I have an evolved state of intelligence, but I would be completely baffled if I had the sole responsibility of assembling the beautiful children that I am fortunate to have. I am eternally grateful that there is a governing intelligence that's giving order to all of the miracles in our lives.

Now, are you living the life that you are truly meant to live? You really need to ask yourself this question and be honest. And *listen* when the answer comes. If you don't believe in anything, you are still going to pick something up. Even if you think it's just that voice in your head, it is still coming from this infinite field of possibility. No matter what you may "think." The poetic beauty of it all is that the source of all of this has now given us the tools and technology to understand that *your thoughts are actually measurable, radiant energy.* What you think sends out a signal, and it attracts back to you what is in vibrational resonance with that same frequency.

Like attracts like. You may have heard this in certain classes and books you may have read; now you get to see it consciously in your own life. And everything that you've ever experienced in your classes and education was *itself* based upon your thoughts; it was based entirely upon your perception, and your individual view of the world.

So where do your thoughts really come from? No one can even see them but you. What about your dreams, your visions, your imagination? No one can see them either, except for you. It's all within you. You can't explain it. And it's not your job to. You just need to relearn to truly *listen,* and take action on living the life that is calling on you from your inner regions to be great! Everyone has that "driving force." It is simply your job to be open and receptive to it. To get out of the tribal mind-set and to achieve the things that you are here to achieve. *Never letting anything stop you no matter what!*

Understand, when I talk about listening, I'm talking about a deep listening, with the *inner* ear; a deep listening from your soul faculty. I'm talking about listening with a peaked attentiveness to pick up on the information that you are wanting to receive. You've got to get out of limiting yourself to the ordinary use of a single sense perception that the rest of society has disseminated to you as the only way to listen. Even your skin has receptor sites known as *Pacinian corpuscles* that pick up sound and vibration, in essence allowing your skin to hear. There is so much more to reality than what you've been privy to, so never limit yourself! There is limitless possibility, and you are the vessel for it to come through.

When you get in alignment with your true self, through right nutrition, right thinking, right relationships, and right living, you will begin to see that the apparent forces that were there to stop you, or to inhibit your progress, will automatically begin to dissolve. You will begin to see very clearly that the illusions that labeled you as less-than, and seemed to be keeping you from manifesting your dreams and living the life that you were meant to live, were infinitesimally small to you. Some of the greatest minds of our time and throughout history, some of the greatest teachers, books, and traditions might bargain to say that the borders were never even there in the first place; it was all within you. It was simply your ability to *realize* that it was there within yourself all along.

Make a Clear Decision

Most people are completely unaware of what they really want. They don't know what their purpose is; they don't know why they're here; they don't know what they are supposed to be doing with their life. It is a simple launch-pad moment when you ask yourself or anyone else: *If you don't know what you really want, then how are you ever going to have it?*

Since most people don't know what they want, they automatically shift to the default plan, which is basically picking up on someone else's idea of what life is supposed to be. This causes a great amount of suffering in individuals. You see this happening all the time now. This is why individuals tend to do what their friends and family do, even if it's not making them happy. They dumb themselves down and put themselves in a box because they don't want to disappoint anybody, they don't want to go against the status quo, and most of all, they don't want to fail. This limited thinking is *exactly* what inhibits you. This and only this is what keeps you from greatness. Understand very clearly that if you are not happy, then you are out of alignment with your soul. Nothing else matters! So if you don't know what it is that you truly want in your life, and what actions to take to get there, then the simple solution for you to do right now is to take a moment and *ASK!*

The Key to Quantum Health

In nearly all great spiritual teachings that I've come across, this has been repeated over and over again in one form or another.

Ask and you shall receive.

Now me being one of the most logical people on the planet, in my opinion, I really needed to see some science on this, because "asking and receiving" just didn't make any sense to me. And then lo and behold, that science showed up for me (I had already asked and received and didn't even know it). This is what brought me into studying quantum mechanics, metaphysics, and the way that things actually work.

Let me explain to you precisely what *Ask and you shall receive* actually means, so that we can get a powerful click to happen in you. It simply means that when you ask a question, you become more *receptive* to the answer that is within you already. You are intrinsically connected to it. It doesn't get mailed to you from some mystical land. The divine has downloaded every single thing that you need to fulfill your infinite potential into you already. It's who you are. You really don't have to worry about that. The answer is within you already, but somehow or another (and you don't have to worry about how), you have hidden it from yourself. All you have to do is ask to see it, and all of the "cobwebs" will automatically be cleared up for you. I know this for certain.

Even if you have the strongest faith in the world, or if you believe you have no faith at all, the surface mind can't wrap around this one. We are talking about pure ever expanding consciousness here.

People say that they have faith, but they don't believe in themselves. People say that they don't have faith, but they are open and receptive to inspiration and ideas coming from "out of the blue." The most intelligent thing would be to liberate ourselves from the impractical games that we play. Be honest with yourself and everyone else around you. If you can't be completely honest with yourself, then who else can you be honest with? We are all infinite beings literally connected to one another, as well as everything else in this energy field that is beyond the scope of the surface mind.

Here's the thing, if you can imagine it, then it's already too small. Your thoughts become the things in your life. This is going on whether you accept it or not, whether you understand it or not. We have been given this incredible gift called the imagination and the ability to think beyond circumstances and manifest a reality that is called upon by our dominant thought processes. The great success teacher Napoleon Hill stated in his classic book, *Think and Grow Rich,* "You have *absolute control* over but one thing, and that is your thoughts." You have the ability to consciously choose your thoughts and even your underlying thought patterns. This is what it means to be made in the image and likeness of the creative source. Your source is pure spirit; everything that is, and beyond. You are that too. You must be like what you came from. Seeds reproduce after their kind.

You, like no other sentient being, have the ability to choose your thoughts, and in doing so, to create the life experience that you are here to create. We have to stop being afraid of that. We have to stop listening to the people that have been telling us since we arrived here that we are separate, and to look to something outside of ourselves for the answers. We are swimming in all of the answers… We are intrinsically connected to it…We are it. There is *nothing* outside of it. We simply need to understand this, respect this, and begin nurturing this precious gift that we have been given.

Simply begin practicing the exercises on the following pages, or other inner development practices that elevate your mind and your ability to focus. By practicing these techniques on a daily basis, you will see very quickly that all of creation is literally conspiring to assist you. That's why you are here, to realize this potential, and to be the embodiment of it here, *now*, in this very moment.

Powerful Practice

Sit quietly with your back in a straight position (either on the floor or in a chair with your feet flat on the floor). Now, close your eyes and focus quietly on your breath. Just sit and watch your breath with your awareness and begin to steady your breath, breathing in through your nose for a count of 8 (filling your diaphragm). Hold the air in for a count of 5 and then release the air slowly out through your nose for a count of 8 (releasing all of the air from your lungs). Now hold the air out of your body for a count of 5 before breathing in again and repeating the process.

Just keep bringing your attention to your breath, watching it move in and out of your body. Do this for a couple of minutes or more, whatever you're comfortable with. You are going to find this to be very calming, relaxing, and quite enjoyable. It is the space between the breaths that is most important here because your TPS (Thoughts Per Second) drops significantly, and you are able to access a heightened state of clarity. Now simply ask your question.

You can ask questions like:
 What is it that I want?
 What is it that I'm here to do?
 What do I need to do to experience the success I want in my life?
 How can I be of greater service?

Or phrase it in statement form like:
   Let me see the prosperity that I am.
   Let me see the peace that I am.
   Let me see the courage that I am.
   Let me see the beauty and vibrant health that I am.

Then finish your question or statement with:
   Let me see it.
   Let me be it.
   I am *willing* to be it.

Then see yourself surrounded by the conditions that you wish to produce in your life, and give gratitude for this experience.

Continuously practice deep listening. Be attentive, because by asking these powerful questions, you've set things in motion to have the answers show up for you. From what I've seen, they tend to show up in the most unexpected, and sometimes unexplainable ways; always miraculous; always awe-inspiring.

Additionally, in this relaxed state you can simply visualize how you want your day to go; or you can visualize your ideal life with powerful sensory detail; or you can visualize anything and everything that you want to achieve in your life. The possibilities are endless.

Asking the Right Questions

Unconsciously, we are usually going around asking the *wrong* questions our entire lives. Question like, "Why me?" "Why does this have to happen to me?" "Why did they do this to me?" "What did I do to deserve this?" And other disempowering questions of this nature.

It is in these times when we feel the most troubled and disconnected (which you never really are) that we need to have the resolve to sit, be still, breathe, and ask empowering questions like, "What is it that I need to learn from this situation?" "What quality needs to be developed in me?" "How do I need to grow to receive the results that I want to have in my life?"

Your focused attention on your breathing is to connect to the present moment, which is where all of your power actually is. You can't breathe in the past, and you can't breathe in the future. Consciously focusing on your breathing instantly connects you to the present.

Banish disempowering questions from your mind. Asking "Why me?" you get more answers and life circumstances as to "Why you?!" If you don't wake up and grow from the circumstances that are in front of you that you may be unhappy with, then there is no one to hold responsible but yourself for not grabbing the opportunity to change and develop. It's simply a matter of understanding that all of the choices and solutions are within you already.

If you choose not to ask empowering questions, and to not take the necessary action towards creating change in your life, then there is only one person that you need to take it up with, and that person is reading this page right now, and already knows exactly what to do.

> *"Always the beautiful answer*
> *who asks a more beautiful question."*
> —E.E. Cummings

> *"Sow a thought and you reap an action; sow an act and you*
> *reap a habit; sow a habit and you reap a character;*
> *sow a character and you reap a destiny."*
> —Ralph Waldo Emerson

Visualization Practice: CREATION STATION

Sit in a comfortable position with your back straight and your eyes closed.

Begin the breathing practice as mentioned in the *Powerful Practice;* bringing your attention to your breath, watching it as it travels in and out of your body.

Now as you begin to settle in, it is time to "tune in" to your Creation Station. Bring your awareness to the outward faculty of your pineal gland, or what is referred to as your Third Eye, which is located between your eyebrows in the center of your forehead. This is essential, because it is from the pineal gland that your thoughts and images are projected outward, similar in nature to that of a projector and a movie screen.

Now bring up a background image in your mind and focus it out in front of you, as though you were about to watch a movie. This background can be a clear blue sky with a couple of clouds, an ocean setting with an endless horizon, a beautiful green field, a waterfall, or anything that feels good to you.

After you have your background up; begin to place images upon it that you would most like to experience in your life. It could be a home, a car, a career, wealth, a piece of artwork, or anything of the material nature. Or it can even be relationships, images of you giving and creating opportunities to assist others, harmonious family events, world travels. It can be anything that feels good to you. See yourself participating in these things; it needs to be sensory detailed, and something that *really* sparks your emotion. See clearly that it is you experiencing these things *now. Feel the feelings that these things are already happening.* (This is very powerful!) You can run these things on your creation station like a mental movie.

Have fun with this! This is where things have been created for thousands of years. Everything comes from the realm of *ideas.* So when you close up your creation station, give gratitude and go into the rest of your day *knowing* that it is already done.

Where It All Comes From

You see, most people never actually experience the world as it really is; they experience their "perception" of the world. It is your *thoughts* and *images* of the world that you are actually experiencing. You are actually projecting your thoughts "out there," and in fact, everything you are experiencing is really going on within you. So as you begin to *choose* what is placed upon your mental movie screen, then that is what will intrinsically become your ultimate reality.

There are several other faculties of the mind that come into play here, like the Reticular Cortex and the Reticular Activating System (or RAS) that literally have magnetic and electromagnetic drawing powers that attract these images *that you choose* into your life. Though this information has been known for thousands of years, it has only recently been confirmed through our leading-edge sciences. It is simply that individuals have been unaware of their ability to participate in this ever-expanding process, and subsequently they will continuously project *and reproject* what society has deemed to be popular, or possible for one's life.

Undoubtedly, you will *always* live the life that you believe. This is fact. Your life is exactly the way you believe it is. You will inherently know this to be true because it is *your life.*

You quite literally have to see it in your mind *first* before you can do anything. This is a powerful truth. There is truly nothing more important than implementing a meditation practice, because this is where your life is actually created. It is from the realm of ideas that all things come into physical form. Everything that is surrounding you right now was once somebody's idea. The seat you are sitting on, the walls around you, the buildings, this book, the words on this page, etc., they all came from the realm of ideas. We've just taken for granted how things work. But the beauty is that now you are reconnecting to the divine structure of things with astonishing speed as you read further, and taking action towards living the life that you are meant to live. You attracted this book into your life. There are no accidents at all. Everything is for the greater good, and for the unfoldment of what Ralph Waldo Emerson would call your *Over-soul*.

The frequency that you put out will set in motion a shift in the course of events that you are manifesting in your life instantaneously. You've got to do your inner work first. And if anything, even at the most microscopic level, if you do these meditation practices with intention, you will trigger your body to release powerful endorphins and enkephalines, which are known as the "feel good" hormones. They are always there and available for you to access to get yourself into the right state to live life with passion, enthusiasm, and a zest for life that is unshakable by anyone.

> *"Your outer world is a reflection of your inner world."*
> —The Law of Correspondence

The Golden Ticket

Here is your invitation into empowered thinking through the power of incredible nutrition!

The following transitional information is simply a bridge. It is a bridge away from all of the artificial, over-processed, lifeless, toxic, fat-generating foods that have been preventing much of society from achieving the vibrant health and physical fitness that we are truly meant to have. As soon as you put *anything* into your system, it sends information directly to your brain that subsequently dictates what happens with your body, as well as what happens with the expression of your consciousness.

Please be reminded that *this is not a diet!* There isn't any diet that is going to provide you with this kind of information. There isn't any diet that is going to deliver you straight truths. This book is a bridge to success, it is a bridge to a higher state of consciousness, and it is a bridge to eating the *best food ever!*

Whatever your particular health goals may be, this information is a bridge to the realization of those goals. So in order to increase your awareness of what kind of foods you have been eating, and what kind of foods are going to send you directly to having the health and the body that you truly desire, it is *essential* that you understand what it is that you actually need from the food that you eat, what you are getting, and where you are getting it from.

Our recent history has seen us become more and more detached from our source and supply of food, as well as the results that food has on our mind and body. We have seen addictions rise and health plummet. So we will begin at the ultimate place…we will begin with where you actually get your energy. We will take this starting point, and follow it directly to looking and feeling the best you ever have! Have fun with this! Be truly excited, because the results that you have always wanted are truly happening now!

SECTION

The Power of Right Nutrition

CHAPTER 8

Enzymes Reloaded

Enzymes are a key component in the actual "Life-Force Energy" found in food, as well as in ourselves. Enzymes are one of the essential reasons that we need outside nourishment for our bodies to function at their optimal level. They are the actual catalysts that provide our body with energy. *Living and raw foods are the only foods that contain the complete enzymatic structures found in foodstuffs.* Cooking our food destroys the molecular structure and eliminates up to 100% of the enzymes that are in those foods.

There are 3 categories of enzymes:
1. Digestive enzymes
2. Metabolic enzymes
3. Food enzymes

When cooked food is consumed, the body is put under an enormous amount of stress because it has to pool its own resources to try and build the enzymes that are absent in the food. Over time this causes excessive toxicity in the body. This is also the reason you often feel tired or sleepy after consuming a meal of cooked food. The body has to take energy away from many other vital functions to try and break down the dead food that was put into it, merely so that it can survive at very base levels of functioning. When the body is put under this constant stress day after day, this greatly accelerates the aging process.

From Encarta World Dictionary:
en·zyme [en-zahym] (*plural* en·zymes) noun
Definition: protein controlling biochemical reactions: any complex chemical produced by living cells that is a biochemical catalyst

As stated in the above definition, a biochemical reaction essentially includes *every single thing that the body does*. Things such as your heart beating, your brain functioning, your lungs working, to things such as your skin regenerating, your muscles repairing, and your body being able to fend of disease and illness, are all determined directly by the amount of enzymes that are present in your body. Enzymes are the very means by which your body does everything that it does. Without the proper supply of enzymes, you are definitely on your way to an early checkout date.

The most important thing to understand is that the definition clearly says **living cells.** You get enzymes from *living* foods. Now, how critical is that piece of information to have?! And it is something that most people are completely unaware of. Enzymes actually deliver the vitamins and minerals (which create your physical beauty), and the other constituents of life where they need to go to do their job. Without them, you become deficient. Deficiency is the precursor for basically all sickness, disease, and overall physical and mental degeneration—otherwise known as aging.

Cooking food also denatures proteins, fats, sugars, vitamins, and minerals; thus rendering the majority of them virtually useless to the body. This is the biggest underlying reason why people often consume more food than they actually need, or even want, simply because they are not getting the actual nourishment from the food that they are trying to get it from. So they eat and eat and eat until their stomachs are so full that they can't get anything else in there. Your stomach itself should be the *last* signal of feeling satiated. Instead, when you are eating nourishing, enzyme-rich food, it will signal your entire body (not just your stomach) that you are satisfied, energized, and feeling amazing. Most importantly, you don't feel like you have a ton of bricks in your belly, weighing you down and making you feel sleepy, lethargic, and energy-deprived.

Again, this whole process puts an enormous strain on your body. You've already seen the evidence for yourself on countless occasions. When you eat a heavy meal of cooked food, your energy levels go down, and you just don't feel that great. *If you want to feel your best, then you have to put the best things into your body.* There is really no other way around it. It's not complicated stuff. There are no magic tricks to having the body you want to have and feeling the way you want to feel. And the most remarkable news is that you have gained this knowledge, and the best food on the planet is available to you now in ways and quantities that have never been seen before throughout our documented history. When you experience the best food ever, *you will know the difference,* and the new and improved you will manifest through your active contribution into you becoming the best that you can possibly be.

> *"As enzymes form the fundamental basis of nutrition, they should have our first consideration in the choice of our food."*
> —Dr. Norman W. Walker

> *"For I tell you truly, live only by the fire of life, and prepare not your foods with the fire of death, which kills your foods, your bodies and your souls also."*
> —Jesus the Christ
> The Essene Gospel of Peace

CHAPTER 9

What Organic Really Means

When a product is labeled *Certified Organic* that means it was grown without the use of pesticides, fungicides, herbicides, synthetic fertilizers, and other chemicals that are scientifically proven to be toxic and damaging to the body. *For a pesticide to even be effective against the pest that it is trying to kill, it has to be toxic; it has to be poisonous.* Because pesticides are poisonous, they are also harmful to humans, animals, and the environment. If you are eating any product that is not labeled *Certified Organic,* or if you didn't grow that food yourself, then it's more than likely that these nefarious substances are in your food, getting in your body, and causing you significant damage.

Some possible side effects of pesticides are:
- Headaches
- Nausea
- Muscle Weakness
- Fatigue
- Respiratory Depression
- Vomiting
- Nervous System Depression
- Numbness
- Diarrhea
- Seizures
- Itching, Burning, Tingling of Skin
- Loss of Consciousness

Sounds like a drug commercial, doesn't it? If you're not eating organic foods, then you're regularly ingesting these synthetic "drugs" that are actually intended to be highly lethal. They are theoretically supposed to be lethal to insects that have been outnumbering humans since the beginning of time, and the irony of the situation is that these insects will likely continue to be around, even if we're not. There is a simple equation for any nefarious substance:

$$Toxicity \times Exposure = Hazard$$

Simply stated, the more frequently you allow these toxic substances in your body, the more likely you are to encounter one or more of those not-so-pleasant experiences from the list above.

Another important factor about *Certified Organic* products is that these foods cannot be produced by using genetic modification or genetically modified organisms (GMO's). The debate on the safety of genetically engineering food has been raging for quite some time now. But most people never even hear about it. The emergence of new viruses, cancers, birth defects, chronic illnesses, and the growing number of extinct species are just some of the fallout being seen behind what many experts call "The Single Greatest Threat to Humankind."

"The new genetic science raises more troubling issues than any other technological revolution in history. In reprogramming the genetic code of life, do we risk a fatal interruption of millions of years of evolutionary development? Might not the artificial creation of life spell the end of the natural world?...Will the creation, mass production, and wholesale release of thousands of genetically engineered life forms...cause irreversible damage to the biosphere, making genetic pollution an even greater threat to the planet than nuclear or petrochemical pollution?"

—Jeremy Rifkin, The Biotech Century

What Do You Invest In?

Most people have never considered why organic foods are more expensive than the conventional or industrial versions of those same foods. First of all, you have to understand that the few extra dollars that you are spending on groceries is an *investment in you!* You're investing in the sustainability of your health, and the health of your loved ones. If you feel good, and if you feel healthy, you will automatically be better and more productive in the means in which you make your money. You will have more energy, more clarity, more creativity, and focus. You will achieve more, have more success in your life, and as a result, make *more* money. It is inevitable.

If you're walking around feeling bad all the time, and expressing low energy, then you're going to feel as though you always have to struggle to make something good happen in your life. And let's face it, that just doesn't make any logical sense. So the first thing that you need to understand is that eating organic is an investment in you. We spend money on cars, clothes, gym memberships, getting haircuts, nails done, countless skin care products, perfumes and colognes. We spend so much time and money to make the outside of our bodies look good... *But isn't the inside more important?*

One more important factor to realize is that in this day and age, when factory farms (who are typically receiving large government subsidies) have a strong-arm on the economic marketplace; it simply costs more for organic farmers to do things the right way. The cost is subsequently turned over to the consumer. This is the bottom-line reason why organic foods cost more; it's simply cheaper to ship the public deficient, substandard products.

On the brighter side, as more and more people are disconnecting themselves from the hazards of the **S**tandard **A**merican **D**iet and starting to feed their family what they know to be the safest, healthiest, ecologically sustainable foods on the planet, a greater demand for organic products is being created. The resulting demand will inevitably create a greater supply through an increased adherence to the organic standards. This shift in the marketplace will unquestionably result in decreased prices for organic food products. This is the way that markets work. You support organic farmers, you invest in your health and the health of your family, and things will change for the better.

This is a fact.

Last, but not least, the greatest thing about organic food is that *it actually tastes better!* If you take a fresh organic orange and put it up against a chemically treated, genetically modified, dyed (yes they do actually dye oranges orange) conventional orange, which one do you think is going to get your stamp of approval? And the same thing goes for all other organic produce versus their "conventional" counterparts.

One more added bonus: *Organic produce is higher in vitamins, minerals, enzymes, phytonutrients, etc.* I often hear that this fact has not been proven, and that this is just an assumption. Well, to quickly clear up this debate, Dr. Werner Schuphan, Director of Germany's Federal Institute for Research and Quality in Plant Production, published his findings based on a 12-year comprehensive study proving the significance of the impact that organically raised food had on human nutrition after *36 years* of comparing the soils and plant products of chemically treated versus organic composting methods.

Schuphan's results were definite and scrupulous. The results showed without a doubt that organic foods are nutritionally superior to foods grown conventionally with pesticides and chemicals. The staple foods in his experiments were spinach, Savoy cabbage, lettuce, carrots, celeriac and potatoes. In his own words, Schuphan said, *"Let us draw the most remarkable results to your attention. The most convincing facts are the much higher contents of minerals—with the exception of sodium, due to organic fertilizing (methods). Potassium and iron show the greatest increases overall. Magnesium and calcium were also remarkably increased in Savoy."*

Some of the other results are as follows:
- Organic lettuce contained 15-24% more protein.
- Organic Savoy cabbage contained 33-40% more protein.
- Organic spinach contained 64-78% more vitamin C.
- Organic Savoy cabbage contained 76-91% more vitamin C.

The results on human health were confirmed by a nine-year set of three separate infant feeding experiments. The infants raised on the organic produce had improved health characteristics including increased daily weight gain, higher concentrations of carotene and vitamin C in the blood, greater tolerance to teething, and improved red blood activity.

Some of the most beautiful and brightest children that I've ever seen are being raised on living, organic plant food. You see these kids and you think, *wow! There is something going on with that kid...* They are magnetic, attentive, and incredibly intelligent to the point that you think that they know something that you don't even know. Truly amazing!

For new mothers, soon-to-be mothers, and those wanting to start a family someday, I highly recommend reading *Primal Mothering in a Modern World* by Hygeia Halfmoon. This book contains a lot of incredible insights into reconnecting to the sacredness of Motherhood, and how to raise your child the way that you want to, in the ever-changing dynamics of our world today.

Children are truly our legacy, and they are at the greatest risk for harmful exposure to pesticides and other nefarious substances. It is time for us to take our power back, and understand that we cast our vote with where we spend our dollars. It's time to make an empowered choice, and only purchase the best for our family, our loved ones, and ourselves. We all deserve it.

> *"Keeping your body healthy is an expression of gratitude to the whole cosmos."*
> —Thich Nhat Hanh

CHAPTER 10

Building Your Body with Intelligence

As discussed earlier, everything in the Universe intrinsically carries a certain vibration or frequency along with it. Everything that you put into your body sets in motion an instantaneous chain of events that attracts either rich health, or disease into your life. Everything you've ever eaten has powerfully affected your physical body, the way you think, and the expression of your consciousness. There is truly nothing more sacred, more personal, and more intimate than what you are putting directly in to your body. It is so powerful and direct that it is simply beyond words.

The most intelligent way to understand the whole process is that if you are eating a bunch of dead, lifeless things, then you are inherently creating an environment of death in your system. And subsequently this is the frequency you'll be carrying. It is a Universal Law that *Like Attracts Like*. So you are literally broadcasting for death to move closer to you. Now, common sense would tell you that you probably don't want that energy inside of you. If you are what you eat, then you are making your body into a cemetery; not a place of vibrant life and vitality.

Furthermore, on a physical level, animal products (meat and pasteurized dairy products) are extremely acid forming in the body and contain *zero* amounts of fiber. This means that when you put them into your body, they are very slow to move and generate a heavy amount of stagnation in your system. Studies have shown that when you eat any animal products along with the **S**tandard **A**merican **D**iet, they drag their way through your digestive system for an average of 4 to 7 days, putrefying and becoming rotten. Again, common sense would tell you that you don't want that inside of your body. Nevertheless, the phenomenal, and yet sometimes detrimental world known as "marketing"—the individuals that unconsciously make the decisions for much of society—insist that you don't listen to your common sense, but instead listen to them. *"Hey, you've gotta get your protein, right?"*

Now, let's be honest for a moment. What they are really saying is something more like: "Hey, you've got to contribute to our profits, right? And if you die or get sick in the process, that's just the nature of the business. We already have your kids on board to take your place anyways. Our most popular restaurant mascot is actually a clown! We're still amused about that one! I mean, how much more obvious about a target can we be?! Well anyhow, it's been nice knowing you… Oh, and before you punch out, you should really try some prescription medication. I hear they work wonders…no cures; massive side effects; but definitely wonders. OK, see ya later!"

This is entertaining and all, but this is what's actually going on. And if you don't unplug yourself, along with your family and friends from this system…well, let's just say it's definitely not creating a pretty picture.

The good news in the midst of all this confusion is that with the smallest fundamental understanding of biology and health you get to discover the truth. The real understanding that is actually relevant to any discussion about protein is that *every living cell **is** protein*. That's what protein is. Every *live* food is protein; it's loaded with it. Now in truth, what we really need are amino acids, which actually create the protein structures. The actual understanding to gain here is that when you cook protein, the amino acid profile is destroyed, and it undergoes a process called denaturization. The proteins get clumped together and coagulate, and when eaten the body has to undergo a tremendous amount of stress to try and break down the coagulated, denatured protein substance to salvage something from it.

What's amazing is our society has actually been trying to get by on this stuff. As a matter of fact, we are told by the people that are setting the standards for health and wellness that we are *supposed* to eat this! It's no wonder why so many people are sick and failing at having the health and energy that they want to have. It's no wonder people are not living the quality of life that they truly want to live, and we now have the world's most powerful "sick-care" system.

When people claim that they are getting all of this protein from some baked chicken breast, or pasteurized milk, or whatever; you can now be able to see straight through it, and recognize the truth. It's time to take the blinders off and become an expert on ourselves, because those days of being sick and tired and not living a life that's worthy of us is over. There is so much good here that is waiting to be revealed, and it is literally boundless. True enough, we do need "complete" proteins and the right amino acids to express optimal health for the human body. And definitely is should taste *incredible!* So we are going to bring in the most powerful proteins in the world later on in the Food and Recipe section. So stay tuned, because it only gets better and better!

Here are some additional facts for your friends and family when they want to know what's so different about you and why you are glowing and looking so vibrant and healthy. You can share this information with them, and let them know that you found out some powerful health secrets. Maybe you can save a life. Maybe it's saving yours. Everything in your life always begins with you.

Some Essential Information about Plant Foods compared to Animal Products:

- When you cook any meat, the cells of the animal's tissues are mutated. The definition of a cancer cell is a mutated cell. So one who eats cooked animal flesh is eating cancer in its basic form.
- Simply cooking animal products releases carcinogens (cancer-forming agents) that are then ingested by the person who consumes it.
- Cooked animal products essentially have *no enzymes,* so massive amounts of energy are drained from the body to try and break down the cancerous substance and keep you functioning. This process results in tremendous amounts of toxins being released throughout the entire body and vast amounts of free-radical activity, which accelerates the aging process.
- Because cooking animal products coagulates the amino acid chains found within them, the majority of the protein in animal products cannot even be assimilated by the body. They are instead excreted as toxic waste products or the toxins are stored in your tissues, organs, and fat cells.
- *All **live** plant-based whole foods have bioavailable protein.* The tremendous advantage over animal products is that you get it free from massive amounts of toxins, foreign cholesterol, and excess fat.
- Pound-for-pound, gram-for-gram, and calorie-for-calorie, Spirulina and even bee pollen have tremendously more bioavailable protein than any cooked animal product.
- Broccoli and other cruciferous vegetables have a multitude of antiangiogenesis phytochemicals that are proven to starve off cancer tumors so that they are eliminated without harming your healthy cells.
- Broccoli, kale, and the astonishing Moringa have more bioavailable calcium than pasteurized dairy products. And it is all easily assimilated by the body.

- Because of its highly acidic nature, meat actually pulls calcium out of your bones, which contributes to osteoporosis and a host of other serious health problems.
- Americans are ranked in the top four nations in the world in the consumption of dairy products, and "coincidentally," Americans rank in the top four in the world with the highest rate of osteoporosis.
- All dairy products contain millions of puss cells.
- Animal products are the only dietary source of adverse cholesterol.
- Just one meal of cooked animal products can damage your arteries.
- Meat and dairy consumption are linked to basically every type of cancer, heart disease, diabetes, obesity, liver and gallbladder disease, hypertension, and numerous other disorders and diseases.

> "Nothing will benefit human health and increase chances of survival for life on earth as much as the evolution to a vegetarian diet."
>
> —Albert Einstein

CHAPTER 11

The Most Dangerous Ingredients in Your Groceries

1. **High Fructose Corn Syrup:** This is a highly processed sweetener many nutritionists have deemed *the major culprit in the nation's obesity crisis.* High fructose corn syrup is not absorbed by the body the same way as a natural sugar. It essentially causes your brain function and the secretion of insulin by our pancreas to become disoriented. It also forces the liver to push more fat into the blood stream. What basically happens is our bodies are tricked into wanting to eat more while simultaneously storing more fat. Studies have shown high fructose corn syrup to be one of the main contributing factors of Type II-Adult Onset Diabetes.

2. **Hydrogenated & Partially Hydrogenated Oils:** Also known as Trans Fat. Hydrogenation is the process for making plastic. Food manufacturers actually process the oils to produce a plasticized fat to make the delicate oils harden and stay in their food to extend the products shelf life, add calorie content, and "enhance the flavor" of their food. Hydrogenated oils build plaque in the arteries, raise cholesterol and triglyceride levels (blood fats), and cause massive free radical activity, which accelerates the aging process. Hydrogenated oils are linked to heart disease, cancer, diabetes, birth defects, obesity, strokes, multiple sclerosis, gallstones...the list goes on and on.

3. **MSG (Monosodium Glutamate):** This is a neurotoxin that directly damages nerve cells, often over-stimulating them to the point of death. MSG and other dangerous neurotoxins such as

aspartame are known as *excitotoxins*. They are added to countless foods and beverages to "enhance the flavor" of the over-processed, lifeless foodstuffs. MSG is scientifically proven to cause obesity. It is a highly addictive substance and has been labeled as "Nicotine for Food." But here's the tricky part about MSG, it is legal for manufacturers to hide MSG on product labels under several different ingredient names. Hydrolyzed vegetable protein, textured protein, autolyzed yeast, calcium caseinate, "flavoring," and "spices" are just a portion of the titles used to hide MSG. Countless studies have linked MSG to diabetes, autism, ADHD, migraines, and Alzheimer's disease. What is the commonality of all of these debilitating illnesses? *They are all related to the malfunctioning of your brain.*

The nature of these dangerous food additives can be summarized in one statement: *What's extending the product's shelf life is* **shortening** *ours.*

What is truly staggering is that at least one of these lethal ingredients are added to nearly all conventionally processed, packaged food items. However, as the public's awareness to the debilitating effects of these ingredients has grown, more and more manufacturers are beginning to take them out of their products. But it kind of makes you wonder why they were put in there in the first place? The straightforward answer is: *To get you to buy more of their products.* And it's understandable to a degree, in some aspects. Everybody wants to make some revenue and be successful. But to do it at the expense of millions of people's lives clearly shows the misalignment that our society has been subjected to for many years.

Well, we've been on that train for far too long. It's time to get off immediately, because we know what it's like now. It had to get this severe so that we have a clear reference point as to what we *don't* want. Now it's time for us to become more aware. It's time for us to become more conscious of what we are feeding our family and what we are putting into our bodies.

You Literally Are What You Eat. Once you *truly* understand and activate the power of this, you will instantaneously begin to put the best possible food into your body, begin to live the life you want to live, and to feel the way that you want to feel. Your body is your temple… And it's all that you came here with… So it would be the greatest of all honors to take the absolute best care of it.

> "To keep the body in good health is a duty, for otherwise
> we shall not be able to trim the lamp of wisdom,
> and keep our mind strong and clear.
>
> Water surrounds the lotus flower,
> but does not wet its petals."
>
> —Buddha

CHAPTER 12

Unlocking the Secrets of Water

Everyone's heard all of the news about drinking plenty of water, about drinking eight glasses a day, about staying hydrated, etcetera, etcetera…But why? Why is it so important? And why, even though people know its true, are they still not drinking enough of it?

To put it simply, *people really don't know how important water is.* They don't know *what* water is, what it does, or the dramatic impact and universal accord that it has with the human body. So to take advantage of the real power of it, you first have to know what water truly is.

The scholastic definition of water states that *water is a liquid crystal with a flexible network of prevailing conditions, thus enabling it to be capable of adopting many structural forms.*

This is basically stating that water is extremely adaptable. It adapts and changes in accordance with the environment that it is placed in. Water inherently becomes, and therefore *is*, a reflection of whatever it permeates. Water is actually known as **the universal solvent.** *It is the vehicle through which all biological activity is conducted.* Ultimately, without water, everything begins to decelerate, break down, and cease to exist.

About three-fourths of this entire planet is comprised of water. "Coincidently," nearly three-fourths of the human body is comprised of water as well. Do you think it's just an accident? This statistic alone should suggest to anyone the importance of water. And maybe…just maybe, the amount of water present in a healthy human body, being the same ratio as the amount present in a healthy planet, isn't just a mere coincidence.

Unlocking the Secrets of Water

We are comprised of mostly water, but most people don't drink enough of it... So what's going on inside of our body when there isn't enough fresh water present?

Water helps blood and its components transport oxygen and nutrients, and also remove waste products from our body. An intake of clean, healthy water greatly enhances digestion, nutrient absorption, skin hydration, detoxification, and virtually every single aspect of our health. When you don't consistently replenish your body with new water, naturally the old water in your system becomes sluggish. And because of the many processes that the water has endured, it is full of toxins and waste matter that very much need to be eliminated from your body. If the old water, complete with all of the waste materials, is not removed from your body, then it will obviously be recirculated throughout your system so that your body can complete its many processes in efforts to keep you functioning.

If your body is constantly saturated with old, polluted water, this triggers one of the primary causes of fatigue, physical and mental breakdown, and ultimately disease. Stagnant water breeds pollution. Just leave a glass of water sitting out on your desk all day. Come back and look at all of the things that have been accumulating in that glass. And these are just the things that are observable with the naked eye! Now imagine if we grab a microscope and take another peek... Would you choose to have this stagnant water in your body??? Well, if you're not consistently giving your body fresh-clean water, then this science project you left sitting on your desk is already in you, times ten thousand!

The solution: Drink More Water! It is truly the very essence of life itself.

We were indoctrinated with this idea that water is just H_2O; that it's all the same, and merely some standard chemical combination. When in truth, even at the most fundamental level, water is H_2O *plus* other things dissolved into it. It is a solvent, so it is always integrating itself and uniting with the things that it comes into contact with. On one hand, you could be receiving water that is ripe with the life given minerals derived from the miraculous filtration process of natural springs. Or on another hand, you could be receiving water from off-gassing plastic bottles that photodegrade (broken down by light) that have plastics dissolved right into it. These plastic byproducts are known as *xenoestrogens,* and they mimic the functioning of estrogens in your body by attaching to estrogen receptor sites. These xenoestrogens incorporate themselves into your body fat, resulting in the "stubborn fat" that no matter what you seem to do, you just can't seem to get rid of it. Xenoestrogens also contribute to hyperestrogen related illnesses like breast and cervical cancer, as well as the over-feminization of men: excess body fat, the development of breast tissue, and greatly decreased ability to reproduce.

All of this is determinant upon making the decision of where you are getting your water from. Get educated about what is most important to your health and longevity. I always encourage individuals to seek out natural spring sources in their area. If you set the intention, they will most assuredly show up for you. You can have the freedom of drinking the most ennobled, high energy water in the world and completely rebuild your body to a remarkable stature. Or you can unknowingly be drinking the water that has been disseminated as just some irrelevant substance, and reap those results accordingly.

Please understand, water is not just H_2O, it is a sacred key of life itself. Within seconds the water that you drink becomes your bloodstream. This is sacred. This is vital. Honor yourself by drinking the best water possible, and super-hydrate your system everyday.

The #1 practice in the nutritional regimen of anyone who is seeking extraordinary health and vitality is the consumption of fresh, clean water. Upon rising, drink at least a half liter of fresh, clean water.

Unlocking the Secrets of Water

Here are some valuable bonus facts about water:
1. The most essential element in the functioning of the body's metabolism is water. Your metabolism is basically your body's transformation system, which includes "burning fat" as well as other nutrients for energy. Every process that the body undertakes is conducted in a water solution. The assimilation of enzymes, proteins, hormones, vitamins, minerals, etc., are all determined by the amount of water that is available in your system for accurate processing. Your ability to burn fat is directly determined by the amount of water that you drink.
2. The vast majority of Americans are chronically dehydrated. Not consuming enough water is considered by many health experts to be one of the leading causes of the nation's obesity crisis.
3. The body's thirst and hunger signals are very similar to each other. The average person, who is accustomed to constantly consuming food, is likely to overlook or misread their body's call for water and opt for eating more food instead. This practice actually causes further dehydration, because now even more water is required for processing all of the extra food that has been consumed.
4. Dehydration leads to excess body fat, poor muscle tone and efficiency, decreased digestive function, inferior skin health and complexion, deficiencies of all types, decreased organ function, joint and muscle deterioration, and increased toxicity in the body.
5. The standard city tap water typically has over 75,000 chemicals added to it because (directly speaking) it is recycled toilet water. Many of these chemicals are proven to be poisonous and extremely harmful to the human body. Not to mention the recycled toilet water that you'd be consuming cannot be cleared of all of its previous contents no matter what is added to it. Specifically, toilet paper residue and tampon paper residue cannot be separated from the water using the methods that water treatment facilities are currently using. When you drink tap water, you are consuming

significant amounts of chemicals plus the residues from toilet paper and tampons.
6. Chronic dehydration increases with age. Your body's ability to signal thirst greatly diminishes due to water deprivation over an extended period of time. However, it can be totally reversed, and your body's ability to efficiently signal thirst can be restored simply by significantly increasing your water intake.
7. Water retention is actually caused by *not* drinking enough water. The body is retaining water because there is not enough fresh, clean water coming in to it. It is retaining water as a last-ditch effort to keep you functioning. Your body is giving you a warning sign to give it more water, so it can displace the old polluted water that has been circulating in it. Water retention is not a sign to take a "water pill," which actually dehydrates you further and exasperates your condition. If one is overweight, you can be sure that it is due in large part to water retention. Proper hydration is essential to weight loss.
8. Numerous scientific studies have shown that nearly all diseases are directly linked to dehydration. Additionally, studies also show that the reversal of all of these diseases is imminent through increasing one's water intake and the maintenance of proper hydration.

To understand this further is absolutely vital to health and longevity. The body breaks down very quickly without water. Without water, you die. It's as simple as that. This should tell you instinctively that dehydration causes the onset of your body's warning signs, which are *diseases*.

The prefix *dis-* means *not*. In relation to the body, *dis-ease* translates literally to mean a body that is *not* at *ease*. If you "test the waters," and go for a few days without drinking any of it, you will find out quickly the true meaning of *dis-ease*.

It is well documented, and well understood, that you can go weeks, even months without food. But you can only go a few *days* without water. What more evidence do you need? Water keeps you alive! Fresh, clean water ensures that every single thing in your body will be functioning at its highest level of efficiency. So, understand this very clearly:

Water keeps you alive!
It is truly a universal gift...
So drink more of it!!!

"*Water is the driver of nature.*"
—Leonardo da Vinci

"*To understand water is to understand the cosmos, the marvels of nature, and life itself.*"
—Masaru Emoto

CHAPTER 13

Manifesting Physical Beauty

It is such a powerful insight when you realize that *you literally get to create your physical body based upon the foods that you eat and the activities that you participate in*. Every bite you take provides your body with the materials that will be used in the expression of your physical beauty.

Some foods cause the body to become puffy and inflamed, some cause allergic reactions, some make the skin break out, some weaken the strength of the hair and nails, and some pollute the major organs with debris and toxic residues that translate into the outer appearance of an "unhealthy" physical body.

Some foods (which you can describe as *Beauty Foods*) provide the body with essential elements that express themselves as glowing skin, strong hair and nails, toned musculature, sparkling eyes, and an inner cleanliness that translates into an outer appearance of radiant beauty.

Beauty is, indeed, created from the inside out.

Understand, there are certain foods that are *beauty enhancing foods* and there are certain foods that are *beauty degrading foods*. The predominant foods that we've been exposed to in our society are beauty degrading foods. This is an important realization to gain, because becoming aware of what you *don't want* opens you up for recognizing what you *do want*. There is so much abundance in regards to incredible beauty enhancing foods that are available to you now, that heretofore you may not have even been aware of.

We have simply been disseminated a tiny portion of what is real and available for every man, woman, and child to express vibrant health, beauty, and health consciousness. It was just the case before that we were literally eating the same foods every single day, and just slightly different forms of the same old thing.

For example, we may have gone to the store on a past occasion and bought a loaf of white bread. Then we find out that the white bread is bad for us so we switch to wheat bread. Then we find out that the wheat bread isn't good for us either (oh those carbs!) so we switch to the whole wheat pitas, and so on, and so on. So here's the underlying truth and the insight to achieve in this:

All of these foods were still made from the same **one** *food!* They are all made from one product (wheat), and it is simply the different means of processing that determine the end result. Now, I'm not saying that the wheat is unhealthy. It is simply to gain the understanding that the majority of the products on our store shelves are made from the same small handful of foods, and yet there appears to be so much variety.

On the other side of the equation, where truth resides along with vibrant health and beauty, *there are literally over 50,000 different types of foods* that are known and available. And of these 50,000 there are sometimes hundreds and even thousands of different varieties of these foods. For example, there are thousands and thousands of different types of berries. There is a profound statistic that states that you can eat a different food every meal, every day, for the rest of your life, and not even eat 1% of all of the variety that is available. Yet, we as a society have been eating the same 12 to 15 foods every single day, just in slightly different forms, and trying to manifest our beauty from that. It can obviously be regarded as another hamster wheel situation.

Understanding what it means to make your physical body out of the same old foods is paramount, because if you are wanting to manifest greater physical beauty, and you are eating the same old foods over and over again, only in slightly different packages, then you will be limited on how far you can go in the expression of your true potential. This is because your cells actually have the capability of learning, which is referred to as cell memory (which is really governed by the master control—your brain). These cells pass their information on to their offspring (which can be considered your residual self-image).

Your cells analyze and process information from your environment and then make the appropriate responses. It is a community of upwards of 100 trillion cells that are working together in harmony to give you exactly what you order up. If the same information and same materials are continuously being used to manifest your physical experience, then there will be a boundary in the way of uncovering new and greater beauty if there are not new and greater resources provided to the body to create a shift in the way your cells are communicating.

What Determines a Beauty Food

The strongest determinant in whether a food is a beauty enhancing food or a beauty degrading food is the amount of minerals present in that food.

When people see you, they are basically seeing the minerals that you have eaten, or the lack thereof. Certain minerals are known to be *"Beauty Minerals."*

Minerals such as sulfur, silicon, manganese, iron, and zinc are all beauty minerals of the highest order, and when consumed in *raw, plant-based form,* they provide the body with the necessary raw materials to "unlock" and express sometimes dormant (or hidden) beauty attributes.

This is an essential understanding to gain because, as mentioned, these minerals are most readily assimilated in *raw, plant-based form. The bridge between the mineral kingdom and the human body is the bacteria kingdom.*

If you were trying to get the zinc your body needs by sucking on some old coins, you are probably not going to accomplish your mission very efficiently. As a matter of fact, you'd probably be doing yourself more harm than good.

Now I know the previous statement may sound absurd, but most people are under the impression that they can get the minerals and vitamins their body requires by consuming a dead, lifeless pill or supplement.

You can only get this type of nutrition from live foods. This is the reality. To summarize this phenomenon, it is the plant that uptakes the minerals from the soil and creates the resources that are actually digestible by the human body. You simply can't get that in a supplement not giving respect to this process.

If you eat rocks, it's probably going to hurt you. But the plant can digest the rocks (the minerals), and you in turn eat the plant, and get all the good stuff.

Food is only as good as the soil it is grown in. So the more mineralized the soil, the more mineralized the food will be. Even if the food is grown organically (which is light years beyond conventional methods), if it is grown in deficient soil, so too will the food be deficient.

This is where sustainable farming practices come in at, and taking excellent care of the land. Our focus now needs to be shifted towards putting the proper attention into having the best possible soil to grow the best possible food for everyone in our community, as well as for the rest of the planet.

How to get the Most out of Your Beauty Foods

Now even with the understanding that minerals cannot be received optimally from supplements and deficient foods, in the same regard, it has been proven that when you heat any food above 118°F you destroy 60% to 70% of the minerals in that food. If the food is processed with little care to this fact, then what is left is merely a dead/lifeless byproduct that doesn't have any real energy content to do much of anything, because also during the heating process all of the enzymes have been destroyed as well. When you bring this into your body, it has to use *your* energy to do something with it. In essence, it is taking away from you, not giving; and that is out of alignment with our true nature.

Enzymes are another key factor in manifesting beauty. It is an essential part of the *life-force* and *radiance* that you are expressing. Enzymes are what enable the body to do everything that is does. Truly, enzymes are where the Master Key resides in unlocking the dormant health and beauty that may have been covered up by previous detrimental practices, stagnation, and destructive behaviors.

Enzymes come in and get things moving again, in essence breaking up all of the "old stuff" and removing the things that are not you, allowing for your true beauty and radiance to shine freely.

Minerals are what your physical body is made out of, and enzymes are what put the whole show together, allowing for continuous life and a divine flow to happen within you.

Without bringing in the minerals and enzymes that your body requires to express vibrant health, your body is basically being forced to do a patchwork job on you. In this case, your body is forced to use the "old stuff" that might be lying around just to try and keep you together. Even further, your body may be required to leach or "rob" minerals from other parts of your body to aid in the functions that are deemed to be more important at the time.

For example, your body may be requiring calcium to assist in the clotting of your blood. But if you are not bringing in the calcium your body requires in a clean, bioavailable form, it will be forced to leach the calcium from another part of your body. Usually it will be from your bones, beginning with your hips and your spine. This is one of the leading causes of disease in the body such as osteoporosis.

Let's face it, osteoporosis isn't sexy. We're talking about manifesting beauty, but if the body is in a constant state of disease, then it could really care less about revealing your true beauty and vitality.

Understand, it's not just a matter of bringing in calcium, it's a matter of bring in *the right kind of calcium.* Specifically in an organic, plant-based, whole-food form with enzymes intact to continuously give you a net gain and allowing the body to manifest its true potential.

The Skinny on Fats

The final key component to manifesting beauty that I will discuss here is Essential Fatty Acids (or EFA's). Essential Fatty Acids are just that: *essential.* They are essential for creating new healthy tissues, keeping your skin supple and radiant, maintaining a good flow and circulation in basically *all* of the systems of your body, and the most powerful insight to gain about EFA's is that they are vital in creating new neuro-tissue. This is the stuff that makes up your brain! And your brain is what creates your body. Everyone truly needs to understand this.

Your beautiful brain is mostly made of *fat* and *water.* These two substances haven't gotten much respect in our culture, but they definitely will. I have already spoken about water in the previous chapter, and how it has been treated so poorly and even neglected in our society. A great shift now is happening towards a reconnection with water, and that which is most important about our physical body. The other word, "fat" has gotten a bad name in our culture due to the apparent over-abundance of it on most people's bodies, and the public being marketed to as if consuming "fat" was the real culprit.

Fat, consumed in raw plant-based form, comes equipped with an enzyme known as lipase which breaks that fat down and provides the body with an excellent energy source. So understand, *"fats" don't make you "FAT"; excess sugars make you fat.* Point blank. In particular, processed, dead sugars, which are a beauty degrading food of the highest degree. Once consumed, processed sugars instantly begin tearing up the inner network of the body. This is because processed sugars aren't recognized by the body as anything natural or normal, and they don't trigger what is known as an *aliesthetic taste change,* which is basically like a shut-off switch that let's you know that you've had enough. You only get the true aliesthetic taste change when you eat raw and living foods.

This means when you eat processed sugar, you can keep consuming and consuming while your body is jamming the excess sugars into your fat cells in an effort to protect you. All the while, your fat cells are becoming inflamed and puffed up. Not due to the fat, due to the sugars.

Again, it is fats consumed in their *raw, plant-based form* that are highly beneficial. Even so-called "good fats" that are heated above a particular temperature can transmute and become dangerous *trans fatty acids.* And cooked trans fats are, by far, the most detrimental food substance that people are regularly consuming.

For example, we'll go out to the store and buy an Extra Virgin, *Cold-Pressed Olive Oil,* and then we'll turn around and cook it. What sense does that make? We want it as uncooked as possible, and then we cook it because someone told us it was better to cook with.

The EFA's in olive oil are extremely light and heat sensitive. So it should always be bottled in a dark container, and if those oils are exposed to too much light and heat, they can become rancid. Even further, if the oil is heated excessively, especially the Omega 6 fatty acids, they will flip and become harmful trans fatty acids. If you are going to cook with any oil, it would be best to go with coconut oil, because it is exceptionally heat resistant and stable at higher temperatures.

Olive oil, in its raw state, is an extremely potent beauty food. And the rest of the good news is that raw fats and oils are a nutritious, fun, and pleasurable addition to anyone's diet who wants to manifest excellent health and beauty. They can be used as an incredible energy source, topically to nourish the skin, and in conjunction with the other components of manifesting beauty through dynamic nutrition (minerals and enzymes), it is absolutely unlimited how much beauty you can express.

In the next chapter you will be taken into the kingdom of some of the most potent beauty foods, and life-giving foods that the world has ever known. Included in the Bonus section of the book (Bonus 4) are several tables that reveal some of the top-rated beauty foods on the planet. So enjoy the rest of your journey, and start having fun with your food again!

"Love of beauty is Taste. The creation of beauty is Art."
—Ralph Waldo Emerson

CHAPTER 14

Welcome to the World of Superfoods!

Superfoods are exactly what the name implies. These are foods with absolutely mind-blowing attributes, flavors, and health benefits that take you way beyond the norm with lightning speed. Some of them you may be familiar with, and they have been available to you for quite some time, but since we have been so busy unconsciously consuming unnatural "popular" foods, we have totally gotten away from taking advantage of their availability to us. Some of these Superfoods you've likely never heard of, but once you start adding them in to your daily regimen, they are literally going to revolutionize your life!

1. **GOJI BERRIES:** These were so unknown several years ago when I first began eating them, that my spell check didn't even have a clue what they were. Now today they are gaining tremendous attention as a powerhouse Superfood, and an unmatched source of nutrition.

   These amazing little berries have been used in Chinese medicine for over 5000 years! That's a long time of documenting anything. Obviously, there is something special and unique about this food. As a matter of fact, it's the #1 Food/Medicine/Herb used in their entire system. It's baffling that we are just now learning about this legendary food, yet because of the unrivaled nutrition that it delivers, it seems to be showing up at the absolute perfect time.

   The Goji Berry is a superfruit that is actually a complete protein! These tiny berries boast 19 amino acids, which is more than nearly all other known foods. They are the #1 source of beta carotene of any fruit (6 times the amount in carrots). They have over 21 trace minerals. And

Welcome to the World of Superfoods!

here's the kicker... *Goji Berries are the only food known that naturally triggers the body to produce Human Growth Hormone!*

Now, to put it simply, we stop producing significant amounts of HGH in our bodies around the age of 20, and then it's typically a downward spiral from there. HGH is basically "the youth hormone," a source of vitality and internal energy. Now you've become aware of the top food in the world that can get those things flowing in you again. *And not only stop the aging process...Reverse it!*

Uses: They are an incredible addition to your smoothies. You can simply eat them by themselves as a snack; toss them in a trail mix, or a salad. You can even make your own Superfood energy bars with the #1 fruit in the world as the top ingredient.

2. **CACAO:** pronounced [ka-kow]: *This is the food that is immediately going to change your life!* This food was actually used as money in many cultures where it was originally grown. I'm talking about some of the most innovative civilizations in our documented history, like the Mayans, the Aztecs, and numerous others. They had gold and silver, they had sacred gems, and they were actually surrounded by precious metals. Nevertheless, they knew that there was something extraordinary about this food. The botanical name of the tree that gives us this food is *Theobroma* Cacao, which translates to mean *"Food of the Gods."* What I am disclosing is probably the biggest secret in the history of food!

Cacao is the seed of a fruit. To be more precise, botanically it is actually a nut. When you crack this nut open, what you find inside is tiny pieces of ***chocolate!***

Cacao is the original food that all chocolate is made from! Now you see this and you might say, "Chocolate? That's not supposed to be healthy. I'm trying to get in the best shape of my life...isn't chocolate bad for me?" The answer is *yes*— if it's the chocolate that we've been exposed to in the past. The boiled-up, roasted, toasted, dyed, dried, fried, chemically treated, pasteurized-homogenized milk added, sugar added, packaged up and marketed to you as junk food or as a delicacy that isn't delicate at all. Chocolate treated like this has become something that is supposed to be a "guilty pleasure." Now you tell me if that sounds healthy.

Cacao is the innocent root of the entire world's chocolate reserve, and it is one of the most nutritious foods on the planet, as you will see. By processing it for mass distribution, over time it has been mutated into something far from its original sacredness. And now it has negative associations with making you fat, making your skin break out, overindulgence, addictions, and *guilt!* No one should ever have to eat and feel guilty about it. That in itself is a destructive process. Massive amounts of research have revealed that the cacao bean is one of the most powerful health foods on the planet. It is the substances added to the chocolate that cause destructive health problems: the dairy products, the sugar, the chemical additives, etc.

The list of *cacao* attributes is simply phenomenal, so get ready because the good news is about to be revealed!

Magnesium is the #1 mineral found in the human heart; and it is the #1 mineral deficiency in this country. Cacao has the highest amount of magnesium of any food, by far! Here's the "magic pill" for that mineral deficiency. Magnesium balances brain chemistry, builds strong bones, and is associated with an overall feeling of well being.

Raw cacao beans have more vitamin C than most berries. It is actually one of the highest Vitamin C foods in the world. Vitamin C is a big factor in your outer appearance of physical beauty.

Now you need to pay very close attention to this one:

Cacao has more antioxidants than any other food on the planet!

Berries, pomegranates, green tea, you name it; combine them all and they still don't equate to what cacao has. It's not even close! The main thing to understand about antioxidants is that they slow down the aging process. So if you want to stay young and vibrant, *eat chocolate*. I know that it may sound crazy, but it's simply the inaccurate programming that we've been exposed to. We've been given deceiving information about this incredible food that *everybody has eaten, and nobody has ever eaten!*

Cacao is literally the most chemically complex food known. Cacao has neurotransmitter modulator agents like: Anandamide (the bliss chemical), Phenylethylamines (PEA, which is an adrenal-related chemical released in the brain when we are in love; this is why chocolate and love have such a strong correlation together), Serotonin (anti-stress neurotransmitter), Tryptophan (anti-depressant amino acid), and the list goes on and on.

This is massively important information that people need to know about. Cacao is actually the #1 weight loss food because it is so nutrient rich. It only takes a small amount to completely satisfy someone on so many levels that it can sustain them for hours.

Uses: You can toss cacao nibs into your smoothies. You can add some in your raw granola or even into tea. You can dip some cacao nibs in a bit of raw honey for a delicious snack. You can put them in the blender with some of your other favorite Superfoods, blend it up, pour it into a mold, and freeze them for an out-of-this-world experience. Or, you can simply eat a few of them by themselves, and experience one of the real gifts that life has to offer. This is all-natural, organic, with no side effects except for *Feeling the Best Ever!*

I've searched around for years to find the greatest Superfoods in the world and the highest quality Cacao products. For more on cacao and how to get your own raw chocolate visit www.TheShawnStevensonModel.com

3. **SPIRULINA:** This food contains one of the most remarkable concentrations of nutrients found in any food. *It is the highest source of protein of any food in the world!* It is as much as 71% digestible protein by weight with all of the essential amino acids it tact! It also contains potent cancer-fighting phytonutrients, such as the antioxidant beta carotene. It has the highest concentration of beta carotene of any food. Spirulina is a complete food source with millions of years of evolutionary information within it. It is a powerful algae that transmutates sunlight into measurable bioavailable nutrition.

   Uses: It's best consumed in powder form; it can be added to fresh juices, smoothies, sprinkled over salads, blended into fresh salad dressings, or whatever else you want to add it in to.

4. **BEE POLLEN:** This is quite possibly the most nutritious food on the planet. It's known to contain every single nutrient that the body needs to survive. *It's beyond a complete protein, containing all 22 known amino acids.* It has a high concentration of the vitamin B family of nutrients, as well as a significant supply of vitamin A, C, D, and E. Bee pollen is a natural energizer for the body. It improves your metabolism, dissolving and flushing fat cells from the body due to its high percentage of lecithin. The list goes on and on! Muhammad Ali was knocking down these power pellets during his championship years. *Float like a butterfly, sting like a bee!*

Uses: Freeze dried or raw wildcrafted is best. It can be added to smoothies, home-made raw granola mix, or it can simply be eaten by itself. Try half of a tablespoon; it has the familiar taste of a crumbly candy.

5. **HEMP SEEDS**: This is an incredible source of protein (35%+ by weight), boasting a full spectrum of amino acids. *Hemp seed is the highest source of edestin, which is known to be the most usable and vital source of protein for the human body.* Hemp seeds also have a remarkable concentration of trace minerals.

Bioavailable sources of Omega 3 fatty acids are critical to human health. Hemp seeds contain a perfect balance of Omega 3's and Omega 6's, which have been shown to aid thermogenesis (fat burning). These tiny little seeds are a tremendous source of omega-3 fatty acids. Omega 3's build cell membranes, which enable them to regenerate and protect your cells from damage.

The majority of the human brain is actually fat! Omega 3's are essential for the functioning and structure of the brain; improving cognition, memory, concentration, mood, the list goes on and on... *it's your brain!* It does everything; and without it, you can do nothing.

Omega 3's are proven to lower cholesterol, destroy certain cancer cells, and improve arthritic conditions. Hemp seeds and hemp protein are one of the new fitness crazes because of their ability to speed the metabolic process and burn more fat.

Uses: You can add hemp seeds to your smoothies, sprinkle over your salads, add to raw granola and desserts, sprinkled over entrees, and make hemp milk. You can also add *Hemp seed oil* to your smoothies, juices, and to even make fresh salad dressings. Hemp is so versatile and easy to add in.

The majority of the remaining Superfoods are given more of a brief summary, but this does not lessen their incredible value. I encourage you to research each and every piece of information that you are interested in, uncertain about, or if only to obtain a greater awareness of your own health. Your level of awareness is the vehicle by which you will receive all of your aspirations (or the lack thereof); determinant upon your underlying mind-set. For the time being, begin to focus on your health. Begin to focus on vitality and longevity. If you keep these thoughts firmly in your mind, and do not waver from them, all of the other pieces will begin to fall into place. That is certainty.

6. **RAW HONEY:** Remember how important enzymes are for every single function of your body? Well, honey is *the most enzyme-active food on the planet!* Add it to smoothies, granola, teas, salad dressing, entrees, etc.

7. **COCONUT WATER:** *This is the #1 source of electrolytes found in nature.* Your body is running on electromagnetic energy. This stuff literally charges you up! It is obtained from *fresh* young coconuts. It has a wide array of vitamins, minerals, and amino acids. The coconut spoon meat inside is incredibly nutritious as well. It contains over 50 different minerals itself. Enjoy coconut water as it is or you can use it as a base for your SuperFood smoothies, soups, kefirs, and more.

8. **NONI:** This powerful fruit is loaded with antioxidants and polysaccharides (long-chain sugars that enhance cellular communication). Noni beverages are powerful elixirs that are created during fermentation, and *known to deliver over 140+ biologically active enzymes to your body.* Try the incredible Raw, Organic Noni beverage *Island Fire* at www.TheShawnStevensonModel.com for an instant recharge to your system. Add a shot to your Goji Berry Tea or mix it in with a few ounces of fresh-made apple juice.

Welcome to the World of Superfoods!

9. **MACA:** This food is the definition of potency. *It is an adaptogen, a hormone regulating food that increases the metabolism, and it is the #1 aphrodisiac in the world!* Basically, it is the #1 food in the world that increases *vitality and vigor.* It's also one of the most mineral-rich foods on the planet. It is extremely nutrient-dense, and rich in amino acids. This is truly some powerful stuff! Add it to drinks, deserts, dressings, or wherever you want to upgrade the power of the meal.

10. **COCONUT OIL:** *This is the #1 anti-viral, anti-microbial, anti-fungal, anti-parasitical substance on the planet.* It basically keeps harmful substances out of your body. Coconut oil also regulates thyroid function, thereby increasing your metabolism. You can add it to drinks, desserts, entrees, teas, and salad dressings…Just add it in. It is also the best thing ever for use as topical nourishment for the skin.

11. **GARLIC:** Raw, organic garlic is said to be *the most powerful herb in the world!* It has incredible medicinal properties: lowers blood pressure, reduces cholesterol, reduces and prevents the growth of cancer cells, kills bacteria, funguses, viruses…The list goes on and on. Most people don't know this incredible fact: Raw, organic garlic also contains a significant amount of Omega 3 fatty acids (EPA). Add some to your raw sauces, salad dressings, and entrees.

12. **BERRIES:** All berries (especially Camu Camu, Acai, Inca, blueberries and mulberries) have an *incredibly high concentration of antioxidants and photonutrients.* Add them to your smoothies, fresh juices, organic/raw desserts, granola, or just eat them by themselves.

13. **QUINOA:** This is known as "the Mother Grain." *It is especially valuable because it is a complete protein grain.* Quinoa is also high in minerals and dietary fiber. Add some to your smoothies, granola, salads, and entrees.

14. **KELP:** *This is an essential for those wanting to balance their metabolism and burn fat!* The reason that many people are struggling with losing fat, besides their overall diet, is because their thyroid isn't functioning properly. Basically, the thyroid gland controls your body's metabolic rate, thus your body's ability to burn fat. This process is heavily determined by the amount of *good* iodine that is available in your system. *Kelp is the #1 source of good iodine,* and it even assist in pushing the *bad* iodine out of your system.

    Kelp also strengthens the immune system and boasts over 50 different mineral and trace minerals. In addition, *dulse, nori, sea lettuce, arame,* and other sea vegetables have tremendous health benefits as well. All of these can be purchased whole or in powder/flaked form like condiments. You can actually substitute powdered kelp for regular table salt and get the good iodine and mineral benefits with your meals.

15. **APPLE CIDER VINEGAR:** Here's one of the most powerful and most widely used substances throughout history. *It is proven to eliminate disease, and keep the body youthful and healthy.* The Babylonians, the Egyptians, the Romans, the Greeks, and in particular Hippocrates, who is known as "The Father of Medicine," used apple cider vinegar for a multitude of purposes, and in particular to treat and cure numerous diseases. We've replaced a tried-and-true staple of our evolution for synthetic medications with massive side effects and absolutely no cures! Apple Cider Vinegar has a proven list of benefits that is far too lengthy for summation. It is highly recommended that you research Apple Cider Vinegar and implement it in your regimen.

16. **WHEATGRASS:** This is highly touted as a virtual "fountain of youth." *One ounce of fresh wheatgrass juice is equivalent in vitamins, minerals, and amino acids to 2 1/2 pounds of green vegetables!* Also included here are the almighty sprouts (sunflower, clover, radish,

broccoli, etc.). If there were one class of food that would be ranked above all others, it would be the grasses and the sprouts. This is a real key to radiant life-force and longevity.

17. **KOMBUCHA:** This is another product that long-lived people have used throughout history, which we are only recently relearning about in our popular culture. It is a remarkable probiotic that cleanses and detoxifies the body. It can provide your body with a powerful energy boost. *Kombucha supports the immune system, increases metabolism, aids in digestion, weight control, and has anti-aging properties.* Organic, raw Kombucha is available as a fermented drink, as a boxed tea product, or the best ever is to grow your own!

18. **MANGOSTEEN:** Known as "The Queen of all Fruits." *This is one of the most potent sources of antioxidants on the planet!* It actually has rare antioxidants known as xanthones that are ultra-effective against free-radical damage. Mangosteen is also one of the most powerful anti-inflammatory substances known and greatly enhances the strength of the immune system. The real magic is in the Mangosteen rind. You want to have it unrefined and unpasteurized, or in a low-temperature dried powder. Add it to your juices and shakes.

19. **ALOE VERA:** This is a very special and sacred food that has been storied throughout the ages. Aloe vera's polysaccharide concentration is absolutely amazing. Polysaccharides are long burning carbohydrates that provide great energy over a long period of time. They are unmatched in there ability to lubricate the joints, brain, digestive system, and the skin. Aloe vera is a key component to any true weight loss and fitness program, because studies show that you can lose weight *and* gain muscle by adding aloe vera into your regimen. Add aloe vera to your amazing Superfood elixirs and blended soups.

20. CELTIC SEA SALT: This is not generally recognized as a food, but it definitely deserves mention on any list of SuperFoods. In particular, Celtic Sea Salt and Himalayan Crystal Salt contain *over 80 minerals* that are all present and vital in the human body. Just to clarify an important difference, "regular" iodized table salt contains an extremely toxic substance called bromine, and it is a cooked denatured salt. This chemically-cleansed sodium chloride table salt is added to virtually every processed food product that you buy! This is the reason doctors tell people to reduce the salt to improve their health. But the thing that most people don't understand, or even most doctors for that matter, is that the most important factor is *where the salt is coming from.*

You see, we need salt a great deal. Salt is actually essential for life. Sodium is the main component in the body's extra cellular fluid. It basically helps carry nutrients into the cells and facilitates numerous bodily functions. Sea salt is a natural source to receive all of the fundamental benefits of sodium, and it is highly cohesive with the human body in its uncooked state. The exact opposite holds true for typical table salt, which is a modern invention, and it is extremely damaging to the body. To put it simply, the body doesn't handle it well, and this is why a multitude of health problems result from the consumption of table salt. To actually improve your health, simply dashing some Celtic Sea Salt or Himalayan Crystal Salt on your food or in your water will give you more minerals than most of the "supplements" you will find on the store shelves.

21. (BONUS) SUN WARRIOR PROTEIN: After being introduced to this product and seeing the absolutely phenomenal results of implementing it into my own nutritional regimen, I would be doing an absolute disservice to everyone not to add this to the list of the world's top SuperFoods. It is, by far, the best protein product I've ever tested, tasted, researched, or recommended, and the scientific data to back it up is simply off the charts. To start with, this is the highest source of digestible protein of any product in a raw, vegan, live, whole-grain, hypo-allergenic, sprouted form. In fact, it contains *85% protein!* It is raw and vegan so you don't have to deal with any of the by-products and harmful effects that animal products have on human health and the environment. It is fermented, so its amino acid profile is highly bioavailable. (This means its digestion and absorption goes way up!) You can't get the type of strength and endurance that you get from Sun Warrior Protein in other protein products like whey and soy. Whey is commonly called "Gas and Blast" by those in the fitness industry, because it usually causes you to feel bloated, gassy and not the best ever. When your system is responding in such a manner, this is a signal there is a problem with digestion and assimilation. If you are not digesting the huge amounts of dead whey, milk, and flesh proteins that you are taking in, then you are overworking your body, getting a net loss, adding to a toxicity overload, and not giving your body what it needs to thrive and create youthful and vibrant health. It's as simple as that.

Sun Warrior Protein uses no chemical additives or chemical processes for extraction. Many protein products on the market use chemicals like hexane in the extraction process. Hexane is produced by the refining of crude oil… this is literally flammable and explosive stuff! You probably don't want that inside your body!

The most impressive and inspiring thing about this product is that it has a 98% correlation to Mother's Milk. This is literally the stuff that life is made of. You are what you eat, and if you are eating foods that create an environment of life, youth and vibrant health in your body, then that is what you will experience. If you are eating dead foods, foods without vital life force energy, chemical additives, pesticides, etc., then what you will experience is a day-by-day decline in your health and well-being, simply by virtue of the choices that you choose to fuel your life on.

To pick up some of these amazing Superfoods, as well as tons of cutting-edge nutrition information visit www.TheShawnStevensonModel.com

Some of the other *incredible* Superfoods that deserve mention and could easily have entire books written about them (many of them already do) are: Chlorella, Blue-Green Algae, Medicinal Mushrooms (especially *Cordyceps,* known as the Mushroom of Strength and *Reishi,* known as the Mushroom of Longevity), and the ground-breaking Marine Phytoplankton. Simply research anything that jumps out at you and take action to create the life that you want to have today.

Enjoy the best food ever! Treat yourself to the absolute best nutrition, best information, the best exercise that **you** enjoy, and the best companionship that exists! Why settle for the second best?! Life is meant to be lived *now,* not somewhere in the future. Tomorrow comes in the form of today. If you are not willing to do the absolute best for **you** right now, then what makes you think that things will change themselves somewhere down the line? *You are the change!* You are the very catalyst to living the life that you want to live right now. If you don't begin living the life that you want to live now then all you are doing, in truth, is creating a bigger and bigger hole to dig yourself out of later; a bigger deficit of health; a bigger deficit of wealth; a bigger deficit in your relationships with your family and friends; and a bigger deficit in fully realizing your highest potential.

Welcome to the World of Superfoods!

Every single person has the ability to wake up to this at any moment. Take action now to live the life that you want to live. No one else can do it for you. Once you take action, you will find that all of the "hard times" and "struggles" that you knew before were merely an illusion, and a false reality that was disseminated to you as the way life is supposed to be. When in fact, you are, and always will be, everything that you could ever possibly want, need, or even imagine.

You have the potential for all things in you. This is a *fact*. It's really about what you choose to focus on right now; what action you take every day in the direction of your goals; and to start manifesting change instead of waiting around for change to come along and happen to you at some time in the future.

> *"Things do not change; we change"*
> —Henry David Thoreau

SECTION

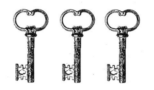

The Power of Bringing It All Together

CHAPTER 15

A Master Key

One of the biggest keys to achieving *immediate* success in whatever endeavor that you are interested in, is so incredibly simple that it's frequently overlooked, and even unknowingly taken for granted. The particular master key that I am speaking of here is to simply go and **Take Action!**

Now, I'm not speaking of necessarily putting 110% effort and focus into your desired result; that would make just too much sense, and make things too easy in the realm of accomplishing goals and fulfilling your unlimited potential. If you take a step back, and look at things honestly from the observer's perspective of your life, you will see that we actually tend to do things very *illogically,* that often lead us to *NOT* achieving our goals in the fashion that we truly desire. This is due in part to our social conditioning and habitual patterns, as well as not having the correct foundational information to apply in the first place. So to begin breaking this pattern apart forever, you want to bring in a real game-changer immediately, and do something powerful starting **right now!**

Speed of implementation is key; and this is what sets apart those who have put success on automatic in their lives, from those who continuously fall short of the successes they desire. Successful people take action, and live in tremendous progress on a day-to-day basis. A typical quality of a successful person is the ability to recognize beneficial information, and to implement it immediately.

It's critical to realize that the underlying mind-set of the *majority* of people is to do the absolute bare minimum in their life. They're just skating by doing the same old things, and wondering why they're getting the

A Master Key

same old results. If you have this minimalist mind-set, then this is the reason why no matter what you seem to do, and no matter what you seem to try, it all tends to fall apart in the end. Because we are usually so immersed in it, we typically can't see what's actually going on. Unless we can take a step back, it's not very easy to see that it was our very own perspective that created the friction for our self in the first place.

On another level you might say to yourself, "I've taken action before and gotten results, but my problem was that I wasn't able to *maintain* the results that I achieved." Understand that this too is because you had a minimalist mind-set at this time.

Most people don't want to admit this, and face up to this self-limiting attitude they are carrying, and this is because it tends to be programmed very deep into our subconscious mind. But just by you putting your awareness on it, it automatically begins to lose power over you. This will enable you to make some simple shifts, and completely release any self-sabotaging behaviors that you are carrying.

You have to put your attention on the behavior that you don't want; forgive yourself; release it; and then implement the behavior that you *do* want in its place. And the secret that is missing in most attempts at behavior change is that *along with the new behavior, you have to connect an* **intense** *amount of pleasure to it, again and again until the new mental grooves are firmly etched into your brain.*

This creates new neuro-associations (connections in your brain). Without doing this consciously, you are continuously going to be running around expressing the same old programming and receiving the same old results.

Why you were unable to *sustain* the results that you achieved before, or unable to achieve a goal that you know you could have accomplished, is simply because unconsciously when you did take an action, it was in an effort to achieve a quick fix, or a "band-aid solution." Those actions that you took did not become a part of you; they were not fully integrated into your system. The minimalist mind-set is always looking for a quick fix, a way to do the minimum, a way to brush off responsibility, *a way to blame others,* a way to benefit without awareness. The minimalist will sit and wait for the arrival of the newest, hottest "magic pill" and will not take the necessary action without some gimmick or some attention-grabber to persuade them. Understand this right now: *there is no magic pill!* It doesn't exist! There isn't a band-aid solution out there that is going to get you where you want to be.

You don't need anything outside of yourself to inspire you. **You are inspiration.** You are literally swimming in possibility—you are made of it. Quantum physics has proven this. Everything is made of energy. Everything is influenced by energy. Everything is interconnected. And what individuals may perceive as material or "solid" things are only tendencies. This is the truth.

Everything in the material world is temporary. And what has been known throughout human history is that energy cannot be created or destroyed; it can only be transformed, or transitioned into something else. These are all-powerful insights to contemplate. Operating in the world from this state of knowing, releases you from the mental confines of what is considered "attainable" or "realistic." If anyone ever tells you to be "realistic," you should make an effort to get as far away from them as possible!

One of the most valuable understandings that can ever be developed is that *everything in the Universe is based on the individual's perception of it.*

A Master Key

You are a creator of your own experience, and it is all based upon your belief structure. You are not "separate" from the field. Indeed, you *are* the field. You are connected to it. There is nothing outside of it, nothing outside of its scope or possibility, and there is nothing that is outside of *your* scope or possibility. Even though there isn't a "magic pill," the good news is that there is a "magic process," and it is called *cultivating your consciousness*.

What's more is this incredible process is only considered "magic" now because you likely didn't realize it fully before. If you were living life much like everyone else (on the default plan), then you didn't recognize the amazing things that happen in your life as a result of achieving a higher state of consciousness.

Consciousness is cultivated through inner exploration, meditation, and practicing the expressive qualities of *The Presence (Love, Peace, Joy, Wisdom, Forgiveness, Compassion, Gratitude)*. Only through cultivating your consciousness can you achieve and *sustain* what you truly want. All of these things have been within you all along. It was only that you didn't look in the place where everything is actually located, to understand how everything really works *fully and completely*. You're beginning the process of unfolding and discovering them now. You simply need to turn within. *You need to do your inner work to see the outer results*. It's not the other way around. When you do this, your belief becomes a knowing. A real conviction is developed that is permanent and unshakable. Which leads to the recognition of this deep-rooted fact: *Your life is exactly the way you believe that it is*.

So what is it that you believe about your life?
I mean *what is it that you **really** believe about your life?*

Explore your web and find out. Face up to any limiting, self-sabotaging beliefs that you are carrying; and replace them with empowering beliefs that you *decide* are truly worthy of you. *See the strength that you **are**, and take powerful action.* What people always seem to miss in this equation is that *you get all the benefits anyway!* It's for you, but it starts with *you* doing your inner work. You simply need to clear out the limiting beliefs that have been holding you back, which then creates the space for what you really want to come in. For more on meditation, visualization, and clearing techniques visit www.TheShawnStevensonModel.com.

Another disempowering programming from our social conditioning is the behavior of frequent and habitual *hesitation*. We have become a nation so engulfed in fear and limitation that we opt for doing nothing, rather than experiencing and taking action towards change. Many people will realize that they are stuck in this reality and take up new excuses like, "It's too late for me," or "I missed out on my opportunity," or "I just don't have the time." You have to understand this very clearly, and understand it with every fiber of your being: *Opportunity Never Stops Knocking!* All we have to do is observe it, accept it, and when it presents itself, *take action!* We tend to just sit around and accumulate choices, instead of acting on just one simple opportunity that the universe has presented to us.

It's time right now to get yourself out of the minimalist mind-set and to focus on abundance and achieving whatever it is that you truly want to achieve. Again, *opportunity never stops knocking!* Now that you are becoming more conscious of this, you will begin to see ever-increasing opportunities presented to you on a regular basis, which can potentially give you something that you truly desire to experience in your life. These things have literally been surrounding you all along; it's simply that your attention may not have been accurately attuned to them before. And how you fulfill this *potential*, is by taking steadfast and immediate action.

A Master Key

As soon as you take action, *potential energy* is transformed into *kinetic energy*, which is the energy of motion. This is not a mere gimmick or slight of tongue, this is a scientific law. As soon as you take any and every action, you set in motion a whole chain of events that will inevitably manifest the "potential" of your action into physical reality. Again, most people tend to sit around and accumulate potential energy and never act on any of it. Thus, by not acting upon your potential energy, it continues to lie dormant, and you never fully realize your infinite nature.

It is never too late to take action. You are never too old or too young to act upon any of the opportunities that are constantly knocking at your door. You are never too late! You need to release that thought from your mind. Do not give energy to the past, and what could have been, or what should have been. Physically you cannot live in the past; you can only live right now in the present. By giving energy to the past, you are living in the past, and you are living in a place where all of your potential energy doesn't even exist. So you are, in essence, wasting all of the immense potential energy that you have within right now.

In the same respect, you also cannot live in the future. You cannot sit around and talk about how things are going to be, and the life that you are going to have someday, without taking some action right now. If you are thinking and talking about how rich you're going to be, how healthy you're going to be, how happy you're going to be, without taking action, then you are just a mere dreamer. Opportunities are always there for you to manifest all of these things, but you have to take some kind of action when they are presented to you, and then *without a doubt* you will experience them.

It is law: *Potential Energy Becomes Kinetic Energy.* When you are working with kinetic energy, then you have set things in motion to inevitably receive what you truly want. Everything in the universe operates according to this, as well as other universal laws. By having these keys in your conscious possession, you become the architect in the creation of your future, and you will be able to enjoy these things in your life right *now*.

All of the choices that you have made in the past have unfolded to create the life that you are experiencing right now; sort of like the unfolding of a beautiful story or a movie. The choices that you make right now will determine how the rest of your story will unfold. Live right now, in the present. Take action right now, and you will see that there is a truly incredible story that unfolds; a story for the ages; a story that will inspire others; a story that will inspire you.

You've been presented with an array of exciting new foods and ideas, and in the next section, you will be provided with a plethora of recipes that can bridge you out of your "old health," directly into experiencing intensely radiant health. All you have to do is try just one. Add something in. If you like it, then add something else in. Just start adding in the good stuff, and pretty soon it will naturally displace all of the "old" stuff. There simply won't be room for it. It will gracefully become an *understanding* that this is the way that things are truly supposed to be.

You are supposed to feel good all the time, you are supposed to be in excellent health, and you are supposed to be happy. When you make something an *understanding*, it becomes part of you. If it is simply a *rule* that you put on yourself, then it is bound to fail. Rules are made to be broken. No one wants to be put into a box and littered with restrictions. It is simply human nature to want to be free. But it is also human nature to do what we know how to do. A better way was not previously known, so naturally we went down the same path as our family, our friends, and society as a whole, which landed most of us in a situation where looking and feeling our best has been a sizeable struggle, or completely foreign all *together*.

A Master Key

But now a new way is known. If you see something that interests you, take action on it! If it's trying one of these recipes, and it's pleasurable to you, and you feel good about it, then it's a win-win. If it works for you, then go ahead and take the next step and try something else. If it's a particular shift in your mental set-up, just try it! Put it into action! If it works for you, then add in something else. Continue to grow. Continue to expand. This is indeed what life is all about.

Whether you understand it or not, everything in the universe is constantly changing. If you resist change, or if you fail to put your energy into change, then your life is built upon resistance, and it will deliver you those results accordingly.

Now is the time to take action!

If you act on just one thing, it is guaranteed that your life will change, and that potential energy will immediately become kinetic energy, which is the energy of motion. When you have the energy of motion working for you, then and only then will you receive what you truly deserve, which is unquestionably the absolute best!

Now It's Time to Eat!

What is provided to you in the following pages are a multitude of incredible recipes that will fuel your path to your desired physical success, and success in life. When you begin to *feel* better; when you begin to *feel* stronger; when you begin to *feel* healthier; when you begin to look and to *feel* the way that you truly want to; *when all of the inevitable results of taking excellent care of yourself begin to show up, the change that's going to take place in your life is going to astonish you and everyone else around you.* When you start to nourish yourself with excellent foods and excellent information, you will undoubtedly begin to radiate excellent beauty. All you have to do is simply let it happen. You can choose *right now* to treat yourself like you deserve to be treated. And don't think for one second that you don't deserve the best!

You do deserve the best. Your family deserves the best. Remember that *you* make all of the choices in your life. You can choose to continue struggling, going down the same path, doing the same things, and (without a doubt) getting the same results. Or you can choose right now to have the life, health, and success that you've always wanted to have. You have the tools now…simply take a few of them and get started. If you want, you can even take the whole toolset! Taking responsibility for your own life and your own health will guide you to the creation of your own tools. These tools will be forever yours to keep and to share with others as you please. When you achieve your vibrant state of health, others are going to be attracted to you. They are going to want to know how you did it. They are going to want to know how this incredible change has happened to you. Share it with them! Share the information! Share the success!

What you are about to create is an infinite state of health, and an infinite state of beauty that will cross barriers where there seemed to be no other way before. You have the fire of infinite potential inside of you.

A Master Key

Release it! Never let anything stop you! You have the *Infinite Internal Motivation* to succeed in whatever it is that you aspire towards.

The keys to your life are in your hand. You are literally creating the vehicle that you're going to take this ride in. Now you get to take full control and masterfully craft your vehicle for this ride. So let's jump on board, start the ignition, and take this all the way to for the ride of your life!

The New and Improved Kitchen Scenery

The essential tools in a raw food kitchen consist of a good chef's knife, cutting board (wood is good), a powerful high speed blender (I recommend the **Vita-Mix®**), and a food processor. With these items, you can literally make thousands of quick and easy recipes, and even gourmet raw food dishes. Raw food is extremely easy to make. A good friend of mine couldn't cook anything to save her life. I mean it; it was like watching someone trying to put a square peg into a triangle hole. She is absolutely brilliant, but the kitchen was like her kryptonite. Then, seemingly out of nowhere she busted out of the gate and on her first crack at making a raw food dish, she mastered her previous limiting belief by making an incredible Raw Lasagna. The irony is so poetic; I am smiling as I am writing this like a proud teacher.

It is truly all about the preparation. Get all of your ingredients out in front of you first, before doing anything else. When you have everything already chopped up, diced, minced, etc., it's as simple as putting it into the blender or food processor and hitting a button to create culinary dishes that would tame the hearts of anyone.

You can go further on your live food creation adventures by enhancing your raw kitchen toolset. You can add in a food dehydrator (I recommend **Excalibur**), spiral slicer (to make noodles from zucchini, squash and other hard veggies), mandolin, and other gadgets to go deeper into the live food lifestyle.

It's just like any other way of being in the world. You create and accommodate your life according to the circumstances and results that you want to achieve. You can do so much with the basic toolset. And I always encourage **everyone** to get a juicer. If I were to pinpoint one single nutritional protocol or practice that has made the biggest impact on my own life, without a doubt it would be juicing. Jack LaLanne and Jay Kordich (The Juice Man) have done as much for the consciousness of those seeking extraordinary health as any other individuals you can name. My gratitude goes to them, as well as to the beautiful Ann Wigmore.

Just as the **S**tandard **A**merican **D**iet and lifestyle witnessed the introduction and onslaught of the microwave, the toaster oven, coffee makers, deep fryers, etc., these pieces of kitchen equipment have become commonplace in the "civilized" home of today. It is simply replacing those things of the life-degrading nature with those extraordinary tools of the life-enhancing nature. Adding to your repertoire of raw food toys is fun, and it's one of those things that you know is benefiting you far more than anything you can even imagine.

You can also add in a magic bullet or coffee grinder for grinding nuts and seeds into fine powders, a cleaver for opening young coconuts with ease, nut milk bags, spouting trays and spouting machines (I honestly feel that sprouting is going to have a big impact on the health of the world). And then you get more into the hard-core live food tools like the mortar and pestle, wooden and glass utensils, ceramic knives, and bamboo *everything*.

In Live Food Living, and expressing phenomenal health, it's all about balance. The real stars of the raw food kitchen are the fruits, vegetables, nuts, seeds, sprouts, sea vegetables, fermented foods, mushrooms, and

A Master Key

Superfoods. The key is finding the balance that works for you. It takes some experimentation and paying attention to how you feel in finding what the best fuel is for your unique body.

All live food is going to provide you with paramount levels of vitality above any dead, processed food. But you want to discover what energetics work best for you over the long run; what foods keep you feeling beyond good, to the levels of absolute unbounded vitality and clarity. You have to experiment and find that out for yourself. Very likely it will change over time, due to seasons, environmental conditions, levels of activity, balancing out deficiencies, and reaching an initial state of homeostasis.

When speaking of the best fuel, foods can be classified into three basic energy classes, which are the *macronutrients:* Carbohydrates, Fats, and Proteins. The incredible difference is that we now have access to the most potent live-food sources of macronutrients in the world, and all are tremendously viable sources of energy. Most people have never even had a real *live* high-protein food in their life. What is provided for you here are the most powerful protein foods on the planet. You have to experiment and find out if that is the best fuel for you. Are you more of a protein type? Is that the best fuel for you, providing you with mental clarity and hours of sustainable energy? Are fats a better source of fuel for you? Is this what keeps you feeling satiated and vibrant, with high levels of energy so that you can accomplish all the things that you want to accomplish every day?

Everyone is different, but you can lean on the side of finding a perfect balance between all of the food classes, which would be as follows:
33.3% Fats (Nuts, Seeds, Fatty Fruits, Coconuts, Oils)
33.3% Protein (Green Leafy Vegetables, Sprouts, Super Algaes)
33.3% Carbohydrates (Sweet Fruits, Dried Superfruits: *Gojis, Inca berries, etc*)

From there you can vary the ratios a bit depending on your desired results. It's important to always pay attention to how you feel, and to understand that if there is a lack of any of these classes of foods, you can become imbalanced, and imbalances create deficiencies.

Maintaining a good ratio of all the classes of live foods provides the body with all of the basic raw materials to facilitate vibrant health and vital energetics. The Live Food lifestyle is about abundance. Over 99% of all the food in the world is living plant food. You get to embark on a journey to discover an endless array of foods and taste sensations, which heretofore you may not have known to exist. Now you get to tune in to the infinite plentitude that life has to offer.

The taste of fresh durian, figs, mangoes, Goji berries, fresh coconut water; creamy macadamia nuts, hemp seeds, Chia seeds, milk thistle, dandelion, fennel, arugula, succulent Greek olives; Inca berries, lychee, papaya, pomegranate, star fruit and cherimoya. Try having a drink with fresh young coconut water, soft coconut spoon meat, Maca, Cacao, cinnamon, and raw honey; it is truly an experience that everyone should be blessed to have.

This isn't even a fraction of a fraction of all the abundance there is. Again, live food is about abundance and having the full embrace of nature itself available to you. It's about taking the limits off and reconnecting to our highest self.

What I have provided here in this book is a series of quick and easy recipes that literally require the bare essentials as far as kitchen equipment to get you started in having the most fun you've ever had and *feeling good all the time!* Most of the recipes shared here only require the use of a blender, and they are all *amazing* to say the least! It's all good, especially when you know that you are truly doing something good for your body, without any side effects except feeling incredible.

A Master Key

Tasting amazing is just the sweet bonus. There are several wonderful Raw Food Recipe Books that are available today. These books often have more elaborate recipes that require some dehydrating from time to time, but the end results are usually well worth it. You can check out some of my favorite books that I recommend in the Resources section. For now, let's begin creating, and I'll be seeing you soon with your new-found phenomenal health.

BREAKFAST

We're going to start at the top with "The Most Important Meal of the Day." The name actually says it all. You are about to *break* your overnight *fast*, during which your body has completed an incredible amount of digestion, detoxification, and healing (especially if you did good things for it the day before). The first thing that you put into your body upon rising has about an 80% stronger effect than anything else that you consume throughout the entire day. To put it simply, what you have when you wake up is the greatest determinant in how your day is going to go! You truly want to reward your body by giving it good nourishment so that it can continue to take good care of you. It is the *Law of Reciprocity;* you get back what you give out. And I'll let you in on little secret: *You really get back so much more!* Now let's get your metabolism rolling with full power!

It's time to blend your way to health, fitness, energy, vitality, success, and having the best day ever!

REAL Protein Power Drink

In a blender:

   12 oz. of Hemp Milk or Almond Milk (Fresh is best or use an organic brand)
   1/2 cup of Goji berries (you can soak them in the milk to rehydrate them)
   1 1/2 cups frozen blueberries
   1 scoop of Sun Warrior Raw Vanilla Protein (Or Vanilla Hemp Protein)
   2 tbsp of flax oil or hemp oil

Blend

(Directions for making fresh nut milk is at the end of the breakfast section)

Strawberry-Banaza

In a Blender:
- Water from one young coconut + coconut spoon meat
- 1 1/2 cups of frozen strawberries
- 1 really ripe banana
- 1 scoop of Sun Warrior Raw Vanilla Protein (Or Vanilla Hemp Protein)
- 2 tbsp of ground milk thistle seeds, ground flax seeds, or hemp seeds

Blender Chef Tip: You can also use coconut oil or coconut butter instead of using the coconut meat inside. Whatever you're into is okay, if you want to mix it up a bit. There is so much nutritive value in the coconut meat inside, and it tastes *amazing* in a smoothie!

Double Chocolate Mylk

(This is only for the true Chocolate Lovers who can handle the electricity!)
- 12 oz. of SuperTea (Yerba Maté, Gynostemma, etc.)
- (Directions for making a SuperTea is at the end of the Breakfast Section)
- 3 tbsp of hemp seeds
- 2 tbsp of cacao powder
- 1 tbsp of cacao nibs
- 1 tbsp of Maca
- 2 tbsp of Raw Honey
- A few dashes of cinnamon
- A pinch of Nutmeg
- A pinch of Celtic sea salt
- A pinch of cayenne pepper

Blend and Party!

Flying High Smoothie

12 oz. of SuperTea (Yerba Maté is great in this drink)
1/2 cup of Goji berries (soaked in the tea for at least 20 minutes)
1 1/2 cups of frozen blueberries
1 1/2 scoops of Sun Warrior Protein (Vanilla or Chocolate)
1 tbsp of Sun Warrior Activated Barley
2 tbsp of hemp seed oil
1 or 2 tbsp of Bee Pollen
A few dashes of cinnamon

Blend

This is what I usually have either before or after my workout. It's great for charging you up or for refueling afterwards. If you are not into flying high, then don't have this drink! This one is *loaded!*

Full Blast Orange Sherbet Smoothie

Hand juice 2 oranges with a citrus juicer and add it to the blender with

1/2 cup of young coconut meat (approx. amount from one coconut)
1/2 cup of Goji berries (soak in the O.J. while preparing the other ingredients)
1 cup of frozen Mango chunks
1 scoop of Sun Warrior Raw Vanilla Protein
2 tbsp of flax seed oil
A pinch of sea salt
A dash of Cayenne pepper (Trust me!)

Blend

The Maca Shake (aka The Fat-Loss Express!)

Water from one young coconut + coconut meat
- 1 1/2 cups of frozen strawberries
- 2 tbsp of Goji Berries
- 1 heaping tbsp of Maca
- 1 heaping tbsp of ground flax seed
- 1 scoop of Sun Warrior Protein (Vanilla or Chocolate)
- 1 tbsp of Coconut Oil
- A few drops of Vanilla Cream Stevia, or 1 tbsp of Yacon Root Syrup or Agave

Blend

Blender Chef Tip: You can also add in some fresh vanilla by scooping out the vanilla inside of the pod. Or if you have a strong enough blender, you can put in pieces of the whole vanilla bean. I highly recommend using some vanilla in drinks, it is highly medicinal, it is a tonic herb, and it tastes amazing.

Optionally you can use a nut milk that you like as the base for this drink instead of the coconut (the best choices are fresh almond milk or hemp milk).

Vita-Blast Smoothie

Hand juice 1 or 2 oranges

Put the fresh O.J. in the blender with
- 2 cups of frozen berries (blueberry and strawberry mix is good)
- 1 or 2 heaping tbsp of Ormus Greens (or another green SuperFood powder).

You can optionally add in some fresh papaya, mango, or a banana.

Blend

Noble Warrior Protein Drink

10 oz. of SuperTea or you can use spring water
1/2 cup of Goji berries (soaked for at least 10 min)
1 1/2 cups frozen blueberries
1 scoop of Sun Warrior Raw Vanilla Protein (Or Vanilla Hemp Protein)
1 tbsp of Ormus Greens
1 to 2 tbsp of hemp oil or flax seed oil
A few drops of Vanilla Cream Stevia or a bit of Yacon Root Syrup
A pinch of sea salt

Blend

Blender Chef Tip: Adding in the power of Alkaline Superfood Powders to your drinks is an incredible strategy to deliver outstanding amounts of nutrients to your body. The Noble Warrior Protein Drink is one of my personal favorites for health, clarity, and sustained energy.

Chocolate Dream

12 oz. of Fresh Almond Milk
1 cup of frozen blueberries
1 half of a ripe avocado (Yes, an avocado!)
2 to 3 tbsp of Cacao powder
1 tbsp of Ormus Greens (or another Superfood Green Powder)
1 scoop of Sun Warrior Vanilla Protein
2 tbsp of Lucuma Powder (or use Mesquite or 1 tbsp of Maca)
2 to 3 tbsp of Agave
A pinch of sea salt

Blend all of the above ingredients adding almond milk as needed to reach the consistency you like. This is creamy chocolaty goodness!

Blender Chef Tip: Adding avocado to smoothies and blended soups gives it an amazing creaminess. The avocado is a fruit that goes well with sweet and savory dishes alike.

WONDER WOMAN Drink

10 oz. of Fresh Almond Milk
1 cup of frozen raspberries and/or Strawberries
2 tbsp of Goji Berries (soaked in the almond milk)
1 scoop of Sun Warrior Raw Vanilla Protein
1 tbsp flax Oil
1 tbsp of coconut oil
Pinch of sea salt

Blend

SUPERMAN Drink

12 oz. of SuperTea or Hemp Milk (Add more as needed)
1 fresh ripe banana
1 cup frozen raspberries
1 scoop of Sun Warrior Vanilla Protein
1 1/2 tbsp of Sun Warrior Activated Barley
1 tbsp of Bee Pollen
2 Tbsp of flax seed oil or hemp oil, and/or 1 tbsp of coconut oil

Blend

Blender Chef Tip: The barley is a great addition to this drink. It's a slow-burning fuel for sustained energy, and has a great concentration of nutrients called beta-glucans that will help keep your immune system like the man of steel.

Raw Muscle Milk

12 oz. of Fresh Hemp Milk
1 scoop of Sun Warrior Vanilla Protein
2 pears peeled, cored, and cubed
1 tbsp of Maca
A few dashes of cinnamon or Vanilla Powder
Pinch of sea salt
1 tbsp of Yacon Root Syrup (best choice) or agave
A few drops of Vanilla Cream Stevia (optional)

Blend

Blender Chef Tip: I wanted to come up with a drink that would knock the artificial muscle shakes out-of-the-park! This is it. It has the high protein power of the Maca and Sun Warrior Protein, and it tastes amazing.

Recee's Peaces Shake

1 to 2 cups of coconut water
2 frozen bananas
1 heaping tbsp of raw almond butter
1 tbsp of Cacao powder
1 tsp Ormus Greens (or another Superfood powder like Sun Is Shining)
1 heaping tbsp of ground flax seed
1/2 tsp cinnamon
2 tbsp of cacao nibs

Process all ingredients in a blender except for the cacao nibs. Add the nibs in last and blend very briefly, or just stir them in to maintain the chocolate chip dynamic. This is Amazing!

Incredible Hulk

12 oz. of spring water
1 1/2 cups of frozen mango chunks
1 ripe banana
1 huge handful of kale
2 tbsp of hemp seeds
1 tbsp of hemp oil
1 tbsp of Ormus Greens
1 tsp of chlorella powder
A few drops of vanilla cream Stevia
A pinch of salt

Blend

Superhero Chocolate Mylk

Water from 1 young coconut + coconut spoon meat
2 tbsp Raw Cacao powder
1 tbsp of Maca
1 tsp of Cordyceps
1/3 cup of raw cashews (soaked)
2 tbsp of Agave Nectar (or Yacon)
A few dashes of cinnamon
Pinch of sea salt

Blend

Some Possible Additional Ingredients are:
- 1 tbsp Raw Mesquite powder
- Vanilla bean seeded (optionally use 1/2 tsp of vanilla extract or vanilla powder)
- 1 tbsp of Ormus Greens

Blender Chef Tip: There are always different amounts of coconut water inside of each young coconut (nature's uniqueness). You can add more coconut water from another young coconut to reach the desired consistency you like. I like my chocolate elixirs thick and rich.

Ultimate Longevity Elixir

12 ounces of Rooibos Tea (or another SuperTea)
1/2 cup of Goji Berries (soaked in the tea)
1 1/2 cup of frozen blueberries
2 tbsp of Raw Cacao Powder
1 tbsp of Cacao nibs
1 tbsp of Maca
1 tsp of Cordyceps
2 tbsp of hemp seeds
1/2 tsp of vanilla powder (and/or 1 tbsp of Carob Powder)
2 to 4 square inch piece of aloe vera gel freshly filleted from the skin
1 tbsp of Raw Honey
A few drops of English Toffee Stevia
Pinch of sea salt

Blend

Blender Chef Tip: You can stir the cacao nibs in last to retain that "chocolate chip" consistency. The Aloe Vera is such a powerful food and it's clinically proven to help you build muscle and lose fat. Incredible!

Banana-Berry Blast

In a Blender:

1 cup frozen blueberries
3 big handfuls of spinach
1 1/2 fresh or frozen bananas (make sure they are very ripe!)
2 tbsp of flax seed oil
1 tsp of Ormus Greens (optional)

Add fresh spring water as needed to reach desired consistency.

This makes an absolute meal! It's loaded with nutrition and it tastes amazing! I was totally shocked how good this was when I first tried it.

Drink of Strength

Water from 2 young coconuts

1 tbsp of Ormus Greens or another green SuperFood powder you like.

Put ingredients into a container with a tight-fitting lid and shake thoroughly.

This is *awesome* after a workout!

Chocolate Icing

10 oz. of Yerba Mate (Add more as needed)

1 cup of frozen strawberries

1/2 cup of mulberries

1 tbsp of tahini

2 tbsp of Cacao powder

2 tbsp of mesquite

1 tsp of Mangosteen powder

(3 capsules of Blue Mangosteen or 1 tbsp of Maca)

1 tbsp of ground flax seed

1 tbsp of coconut oil

1 tsp of raw honey

Blend all of the ingredients adding more tea as needed to reach your desired consistency.

This is one of the best drinks I've ever had! It is literally like delicious Chocolate Icing. Loaded with SuperFoods!

The Chocolate Immortal

12 oz. of SuperTea
4 tbsp of hemp nuts
2 tbsp of Cacao powder
2 tbsp of Lucuma powder
1 to 2 tbsp of Maca
2 tbsp of Tocotrenols
1/4 tsp of cinnamon
1 tbsp of raw honey
2 to 10 capsules of Medicinal Mushrooms (open the capsules and pour them in)
Pinch of sea salt

Blend

Blender Chef Tip: I named this *The Chocolate Immortal* because of all of the powerful anti-aging properties brought in by the Tocotrenols, Cacao, and the Medicinal Mushrooms. Try adding a variety of different Medicinal Mushrooms to this drink. They all have amazing health benefits. This is one of my personal favorites.

Cookies & Cream

1 cup of coconut water + coconut spoon meat
1/2 cup of raw cashews (soaked for at least 4 hours)
1 1/2 tbsp of quinoa flakes (or 2 tbsp of sprouted quinoa)
1 tbsp of ground flax seed
2 tbsp of cacao nibs
1 tsp of raw honey
1 1/2 frozen bananas
Pinch of sea salt

Blend all of the ingredients together. Add more coconut water as needed.

Special Announcement! There really is something about this combination that causes an added feeling of euphoria. It could be the Quinoa (The Mother Grain) and Cacao (The Food of the Gods) coming together and having a good time... *Go ahead and judge for yourself!*

Note: This drink may cause you to have the best day ever!

Recipes

The Chocolate Champion

12 ounces of cold Pau D'arco and Cat's Claw Tea (or another SuperTea)
1 tbsp of coconut oil (or coconut butter)
3 tbsp of hemp seeds
2 tbsp of Cacao Powder (or ground cacao nibs)
1 tbsp of Maca
1 tbsp of Mesquite (or 1/2 tsp of cinnamon)
1 or 2 tbsp of Raw Honey
Medicinal Mushrooms
   (esp. Reishi and Cordyceps; open 2 to 10 capsules and pour them in)

Blend

This is my signature drink. It will literally change your experience of day-to-day life. If you are looking for extreme levels of energy and clarity, it will do that. Because of the MAO inhibitors and many of the other biopotentiator constituents, if you are looking for healing from a particular health condition, it will assist in that too. You can simply alter the ingredients a bit to emphasize your particular situation, and it will literally go to work on you to create the right conditions for healing to manifest with promptness. For example, if you're dealing with a candida situation, you can go with a Pau D'arco tea base and go from there. If you're dealing with cancer, you can load it up with a Medicinal Mushroom complex, providing your body with the tools and information it needs to actually enable you to heal. And guess what? You can actually enjoy getting well! It is truly too simple to express in writing.

Extras

Coconut-Banana Breeze

Crack open a young coconut, pour it into a bender, add a couple of frozen bananas, blend, and presto! Excellent energy. Excellent nutritional benefits.

Some Possible Additional Ingredients are:
- 1/2 cup of Goji berries
- 2 tbsp of hemp seeds
- 2 tbsp of flax oil
- 1 to 2 tbsp of Maca and/ or Cacao nibs
- 1 tbsp of Ormus Greens

Fresh Fruit or Fresh-Made Juice

There isn't a better breakfast than this. There are no rules here…*anything goes!*

Gone Bananas

Slice a banana lengthwise

Spread raw almond butter or cashew butter on top

Sprinkle cacao nibs all over and enjoy!

(My kids love this one.) (You can also sprinkle some hemp nuts on top too.)

Bowl of Magic

Have Goji berries, a diced banana, a tsp of raw honey with several tbsp of cacao nibs and hemp seeds mixed up in a bowl of love. You can even add some fresh nut milk to the mix. Enjoy!

Almond Mylk

1 cup of raw almonds soaked and peeled
3 cups of water
Pinch of Celtic sea salt

Blend ingredients in a blender until smooth and strain through a nut milk bag or cheese cloth. Double or triple the ingredients to make the amount of Mylk that you want. You can flavor the Mylk any way that you like, or leave it plain, refrigerate it, and use it as a base for some incredible drinks. You can make other types of Mylk also: Brazil nut, hemp nut (no soaking needed), etc.

SuperTeas

Medicinal teas have been used for thousands of years to prevent, treat, and cure illnesses. Traditionally teas have been used to amplify energy, enhance mental focus, increase vitality, and to facilitate the health and well-being of the body. Some teas are so powerful and sought-after that they have a special place and sanctity in their particular indigenous culture. What I call SuperTeas are the teas that have powerful qualities beyond "the norm," that can instantly give someone a much-needed upgrade in their health and nutrition.

Teas like Yerba Maté, Gynostemma, Cat's claw, Pau D'arco, Chuchuhuasi, and even Goji Berry Tea are among many of the world-renowned SuperTeas. These incredible teas are an essential and fun part of anyone's nutritional regimen who is seeking extraordinary fitness, clarity, vitality, and wanting to experience the best health ever!

My strategy for making a SuperTea is two basic methods.

Method 1:

Teas like Yerba Maté are extremely high in antioxidants and other incredible vital nutrients that can be damaged in the heating process. So what I do is take the particular tea leaves (or if you are using teabags, that's okay too), add the desired amount of water and warm the tea over very low heat for a longer period of time.

For example: If I want to make 32 oz. of tea to have some for later, I'll take 4 tbsp of tea, add the water, put a lid on the pot, and warm it over very low heat for about 20-30 min (low enough that I can still put my finger in it after it is done brewing, but still hot enough to extract the goodies from the tea leaves). Then I'll simply let it sit for about an hour or so. I'll just bottle it up and refrigerate it to use as a base for making some incredible Superfood Elixirs, Chocolate Mylks, or whatever else I may want. If I want to have a warm tea drink, like a "Hot Chocolate" then I'll simply use it while it's warm, put it in the blender with all of my other SuperFoods, and then blend my way to bliss. It's so simple! You will always find bottles of fresh SuperTeas in my refrigerator, just waiting to become the next SuperFood Elixir.

Method 2:

Teas like Pau D'arco and Cat's claw are barks. They are very tough and resilient, and you do have to cook them down a bit to extract the good stuff to make a powerful tea. My strategy is to take the desired amount of the tea and water and warm it over low heat for about an hour, until the water is just under boiling. Then I'll let it sit for about an hour and then I'll repeat the process again one or even two more times. Bottle it up and use it a base for some of the most powerful healing, life-giving drinks that you can imagine.

Research and experiment with these SuperTeas and you will find yourself disconnecting from so much stagnation and uncertainty, and experiencing levels of health and vitality that heretofore you did not even know existed.

Enjoy!

LUNCH TIME

After lunch is the time when most people slow down, start to feel sluggish, and begin waiting for their day to just be over …

Typically, when you used to eat a heavy meal of cooked food for lunch, your body would have to use its own enzyme stores, or "life-force energy" to break down all of that dead food that you just put into it. Additionally, because we had been eating what is popular, not what's *real*, almost none of the stuff that we've been eating exists anywhere in nature. Putting this lifeless food into your body sets off an immediate immune system response, which again lowers your energy levels because your body is more focused on keeping you alive and cleaning up the mess that was put in to it, than giving you the energy that you require to feel good, work on your gifts and talents, and manifest the life that you truly want to have. We all grew up in a society were it's been accepted as "normal" to keep getting a net loss when we eat…What sense does that make?

But now the good news! Those days are over! You are stepping out of the "normal" paradigm and stepping into what's real; giving your body what it needs to give you the life that you want have. When you eat, you are *supposed* to feel good; you are *supposed* to feel energized. That is the whole purpose of eating; to give your body what it needs to function at its optimum level! After lunch, the day still has so much opportunity. Now let's give your body what it needs to put 110% into whatever it is that you want to experience.

To really stay in the flow, I like to have Superfood Elixir for lunch that has a high concentration of amino acids and minerals; either hemp nuts or Sun Warrior Protein to really power me through the day and evening. Try any of the recipes and even mix it up and create a signature drink that works the best for you. Be an alchemist, and blend your way to phenomenal health. Oh, and most importantly, it has to taste *amazing!*

Here are some great lunch options:

POWER SALADS

Superhero Salad

1 huge bowl of spinach and baby lettuces
1 carrot, shredded
1 tomato, diced
1 avocado, cubed
1/2 tsp of kelp powder
2 tbsp dehydrated pumpkin seeds
Black pepper to taste

DRESSING:

2 tbsp of fresh squeezed lemon
2 tbsp of Apple Cider Vinegar
2 tbsp of Noma Shoyu or wheat-free Tamari
2 tbsp of Extra Virgin Olive Oil
1 tsp fresh garlic (shredded/minced)

For the dressing, mix all ingredients in a cup. Pour it over your salad. Sprinkle the pumpkin seeds on top and dash a little bit of ground black pepper to taste.

Sweetheart Salad

Mixed baby lettuces
1 shredded carrot
1 handful of diced sweet red bell pepper
1 big handful of raw pecans or macadamia nuts
1 handful of raisins
1/2 diced cucumber (optional)
2 tbsp shredded coconut flakes (optional)

For dressing combine

2 tbsp of flax seed oil or hemp oil
Juice from 1/2 orange (fresh-squeezed)

Beauty Salad

Fresh leafy greens of your choice (Be sure to include some Arugula in the mix)
1 avocado, cubed
Radishes (Matchstick sliced)
1 tomato chopped
1 big handful of your favorite sprouts (clover, alfalfa, broccoli, sunflower, etc.)
1 or 2 tbsp dehydrated pumpkin seeds

For dressing combine

2 tbsp of flax seed oil (or another kind)
2 tbsp of Apple Cider Vinegar
1 tbsp of Nama Shoyu or Braggs Liquid Aminos

Sprinkle on some black pepper and about 1 tbsp of dulse or kelp granules.

Recipes

Creamy Kale Salad

1 bunch of kale (shredded)
1 avocado
1 tomato diced
2 tbsp of fresh lemon juice
2 tbsp of hemp oil (or olive oil)
1/2 tsp of Celtic sea salt
1/4 tsp of cayenne pepper

After de-stemming and shredding the kale, add it to a large bowl. To really break down the plant fibers in the kale and really make it manageable and delicious, you need to massage the kale with the sea salt for about 2 minutes or so (massage and squeeze it and will begin to take on a softer look and feel.) Now add in the avocado and continue massaging (That's right! It's time to get your hands in there! Be a kid again, and play with your food! It's going to be so worth it!) Now mix in the other ingredients with a fork or spoon, put it on serving plates, and top with kelp powder and a tbsp of hemp nuts.

Now, I really want to re-emphasize:
I love to stay *in the flow* at lunch time, so what I tend to go for is a Superfood elixir that really caters towards everything that I am needing in the moment to really elevate me to the next level for my day. Of course, the amazing taste sensations are a determining factor! I like to go with a cacao drink for lunch with raw hemp nuts and coconut oil somewhere in the mix. It's really about experimenting and finding out what works best for you. What really enables you to feel the best all the time! This is what's possible. This is where things are truly headed.

ENTREES/DINNER

Here we are at the most controversial meal of the day. You hear various books, articles, and people say things like, "You shouldn't eat after that time" or "You shouldn't eat that for dinner" or "You should watch the amount of _____ that you eat in the evening." Fill in the blank with whatever you want: fat, starches, sugar, calories; it doesn't really matter anyway. True enough, if you're eating a two-piece and a biscuit at midnight, then yes, you're going to pack on some extra fat. But if you're eating nutritious food with actual enzymes, vitamins, minerals, and vital life-force energy, then you can't go wrong! You can eat whatever you want, at whatever time that you want, and feel great! You don't have to live your life being controlled by the clock. You'll actually be surprised how much time you have when you're not worried about time. Let it go and have the best night ever!

Pizza Love

Makes 3 pizzas

FRESH MARINARA SAUCE:

2 medium tomatoes, cubed
8 to 10 sun dried tomatoes (soaked at least 20 min. in spring water)
1 garlic clove
1 tbsp red onion, minced
2 tbsp fresh basil, chopped
1 tsp oregano
1/2 tsp sea salt
1 tsp of raw honey

Place all ingredients in a blender and process, maintaining a thick consistency.

BEAUTIFYING EMERALD "CHEEZE" SAUCE:

1 large avocado

3 tbsp soaking water from sun dried tomatoes

With your food processor or magic bullet, process the avocado with just enough water for it to become a nice, creamy consistency.

PIZZA CRUST and Assembly

Use Flax crackers, Vegetable crackers, Fresh Living Grain Crust, or if you're not going 100% Live for this dish, you can use some Whole Grain Pitas. Place your pizza crust of choice on your plate. Next, spread fresh marinara sauce over it and then carefully spread the avocado over the marinara sauce using the back of the spoon. Finally, top it off with mushrooms, Greek olives, onions, or whatever else you want on your pizza. *That's Amore!*

Stuffed Tomatoes

Makes filling for 5 to 6 tomatoes

CHEEZY PATÉ

1 cup of pistachios

1 cup of sunflower seeds, soaked

1/2 cup of pine nuts

3 tbsp of olive oil (or hemp oil)

1/2 cup tomato "innards" (The inside of one or two of the tomatoes)

1/2 cup lemon juice

1/4 cup water

3 tbsp each of fresh thyme and basil, minced

1/2 tsp Celtic sea salt

Process in a blender or a food processor with an s-blade until you achieve the consistency you like (likely very smooth). Cut out the top of a tomato, scoop out the inside, save to processes into the pate. Fill tomatoes and garnish. As an option, dehydrate on 110°F for two hours to warm.

Easy Nori Rolls

Dried Nori sheets
Avocado sliced lengthwise
Cauliflower (pulsed in a food processor to resemble rice)

Spread ingredients into nori sheets and roll. Serve with Noma Shoyu or another raw dipping sauce.

Note: If you don't have a food processor, you can just chop up the cauliflower very fine by hand. Let nothing stop you from making these tasty treats.

Nori Rules!

Dried Nori sheets
Carrots and Celery (Sliced julienne)
Tomato (sliced julienne with the insides still intact)
Avocado sliced lengthwise
Mock Salmon Paté (see recipe provided. Amazing!)
Alfalfa sprouts
Kelp or Dulse granules

Lay out your nori sheets on a napkin, plate, or sushi mat. Add all of your ingredients onto the nori sheet horizontally on the lower portion of the sheet, leaving about 2 inches at the bottom to roll it up. After layering your ingredients, roll it up, cut it into bit-size "sushi" portions, and serve with your favorite dipping sauce.

Mock Salmon Paté
   2 cups walnuts
   2 stalks celery
   1 large red bell pepper
   1/4 cup red onion
   1 1/2 tsp sea salt

Combine all ingredients in a food processor blend until smooth. Can be served as paté for nori roll, rolled up in a fresh collard leaf, or with flax crackers

Crispy Revolution Pizza Bites
   Hummus (Flax or Zucchini based is best. Matter of Flax makes a good one)
   Shredded lettuce
   Diced tomatoes
   Diced avocado
   Chopped mushrooms
   (and/or olives. Greek and Kalamata are some good choices)

Put all of the ingredients on top of your favorite flax crackers in the order above and enjoy the new pizza revolution!

Taco Salad
   Shredded lettuce
   Diced tomatoes
   Salsa Live! (Recipe Provided)
   The GUAC (Recipe Provided)
   Spicy Walnut Taco Filling (Recipe Provided. Unbelievable!)
   Mexican Style Flax crackers
   The Sour Cream (Recipe Provided)

Layer the ingredients in personal sized bowl from the bottom up like this:
Flax Crackers/Spicy Walnut Taco Filling/Lettuce/Salsa

Then repeat so that you'll have two layers of taco goodness and then top it all off with a heaping tbsp of The GUAC and The Sour Cream.

Salsa Live!

4 medium tomatoes chopped (Place in a bowl and drain away some of the juice)
1/2 jalapeno pepper (or more depending on how hot you like it)
1/2 cup red onion chopped
1/2 cup cilantro (de-stemmed and chopped)
1 garlic clove
2 tbsp of fresh lime juice
Dash of cracked pepper
Sea salt to taste (start with about 1/2 tsp and add more if you like)

In a food processor pulse the jalapeno, garlic, cilantro, and half of the chopped onion. Then add in the tomatoes, lime juice, salt, pepper, and remaining onion.

Process gently now to retain the chunky texture (very important!). Processing it too much will give you a runny consistency. We want it *thick*. Refrigerating it for a couple of hours is a good idea too. If you let it sit for a while, it tastes even better!

The GUAC

In a bowl, add 3 ripe avocadoes with about 3/4 cup of *Salsa Live!* and 1/2 tsp of sea salt. Mash it thoroughly with a fork. That's The GUAC. Yes, it is that easy and so good! You can serve this with flax crackers, chopped veggies, or as a topping for other entrees.

(Optionally, you can do this in the food processor if you like.)

Recipes

Spicy Walnut Taco Filling

1 1/2 cups soaked walnuts
1 tbsp chili powder
1 tbsp cumin
1/4 cup fresh cilantro (de-stemmed and chopped)
1 tsp dried cilantro (coriander)
1 small tomato (diced)
2 tbsp of Braggs Liquid Aminos

Pulse all ingredients in a food processor to achieve a "ground meat" texture.

It is really, really, really like taco "meat," but it is all good! You're getting a rich dose of Omage-3's from the walnuts. Plus enzymes, fiber, and several minerals and trace mineral to top it off (the taco meat that we grew up with is officially retired!)

The Sour Cream

2 cups of cashews (soaked at least 4 hours)
1/2 cup of olive oil
3 to 4 tbsp of lemon juice
1 1/2 tsp of sea salt
3/4 cup of water (add more as needed to reach desired consistency)

My daughter first made this recipe when we were having taco night, and it was sort of at the last minute so I almost told her to just wait and make it another time…Man, I am so glad that I went ahead and let her make this. All I can say is, thank you, Jasne.

Macho Tacos
Spicy Walnut Taco Filling
Salsa Live!
The Guac
The Sour Cream
Purple Cabbage
1 large tomato
Shredded lettuce

Cut the bottom of the cabbage where all of the leaves come together so that you can remove several leaves from it. This will be your purple shell. Fill it up with goodies the way that you like and enjoy!

Cado & Cracker Mini-Sandwiches
Flax crackers
Avocado
Cucumber
Tomato
Cayenne pepper
Sprouts
Kelp granules

Layer the ingredients onto your crackers to make little "sandwiches" in the order above, from top to bottom. Delicious, easy, and a real meal.

Popeye and Olive

   3 cups of spinach

   1 cup of Cheezy Paté (Recipe under *Stuffed Tomatoes*)

   10 to 20 olives pitted and sliced (Greek or Kalamata)

   1 medium tomato diced

   Kelp granules

   Golden Greek Dressing (Recipe Provided in the Dressing Section)

Spread your spinach across a plate, covering the plate entirely. Put a couple of serving of the Cheezy paté on top of the spinach. Next, cover the plate with the diced tomatoes, olives, pour over a bit of Golden Greek and dash some kelp or dulse flakes over the top. Grab a fork, take a bite and watch the smile come up.

Falafel Balls

   2 cups soaked sunflower seeds

   3/4 cup fresh cilantro (de-stemmed and chopped)

   1 tbsp red onion chopped

   2 garlic cloves chopped

   2 tbsp of tahini

   1/2 tsp of cumin

   1/2 cup fresh squeezed lemon juice

   1/4 tsp of sea salt

In a food processor, grind the sunflower seeds into a fine powder. Next, add all the remaining ingredients and process again. After processing, roll the falafel mix into balls about the size of traditional meatballs and sit them on a plate or serving tray.

For those who don't know what falafel is, it is a Middle Eastern dish that is similar to a savory "meatball." This is really, really good.

You can roll these up in a large collard leaf with shredded carrots, tomatoes, raw olives, sprouts, kelp granules, and whatever else you like. You've got to try this one!

LIFE-FORCE BLENDED SOUPS

Life-Force Blended Soups are highly nutritious meals that only require you to put all the ingredients into a blender and hit the button. The taste is the real bar to measure it by. You absolutely have to taste to believe it! These soups are served as is, and only warmed by the processing of the blender to retain all of the vital nutrients and life-force that we want from our food.

Pleasure Soup

1 1/2 cups of spring water
4 tbsp of raw tahini
1/2 cucumber, with peel
1 red pepper, cored and deseeded
1 medium tomato
1/2 cup lemon juice, fresh squeezed
1 tablespoon ginger root, peeled and chopped
2 whole garlic cloves
1/4 cup red onion
1 cup cilantro (fresh)
2 heaping tbsp of unpasteurized brown rice miso
2 tbsp of extra virgin olive oil
1 tbsp Noma Shoyu or Braggs Liquid Aminos
1/4 tsp cayenne pepper
2 tbsp of nutritional yeast (or soy lecithin)
Dash Celtic Sea salt and fresh black pepper to taste

Recipes

Just set all the ingredients out for putting in the blender and this only takes a few minutes to make. The name of the soup says it all!

Cut all of the vegetable into chunks and put all the ingredients in the blender and blend them together. Depending on the size and power of your blender, you may need to stop the blending to push the ingredients down towards the blade and then continue blending until smooth. Or you can blend all of the vegetables with the spring water first and then add the rest of the ingredients.

Serves 2 to 4 (or you can save some for tomorrow's lunch and enjoy it again!)

Fennel Soup

  3 cups chopped fennel
  1 cup of pine nuts (plus a little more)
  1/4 cup of olive oil
  1/2 cup of lemon juice
  1 tsp of Celtic Sea salt
  Dash of white pepper
  1 cup of coconut water (add more as needed to reach desired consistency)

Blend all ingredients in a blender until smooth. Pour into bowls and drizzle over some extra virgin olive oil, then top with a bit of finely chopped basil.

I first had this amazing soup while I was in Miami on my honeymoon. This is the best summer soup ever!

Serves 2

Creamy Broccoli Soup

4 cups chopped broccoli
1 avocado
2 cloves of garlic
2 tbsp of red onion
1 tbsp of raw honey
1 tbsp of olive oil
1/2 tsp of cumin (or more if you like it spicy)
1 tsp of sea salt
Dash of cayenne pepper
1/2 cup of Brazil nuts (soaked at least 4 hours)
3 cups of structured water
1 tbsp of Soy Lecithin (optional)

Blend all ingredients in a blender until smooth and you reach your desired temperature. You can always add a bit more salt and/or cumin if you want to bring the flavors out a bit more.

Note: Optionally, you can use fresh almond milk or Brazil nut milk in place of the water and omit using the actual Brazil nuts in the recipe. That is my favorite way to do it. This is truly one of the best soups ever!

Serves 2

Recipes

Creamy Tomato Soup

   4 medium tomatoes
   1 green pepper, seeded
   1/2 cup sweet yellow onion
   1 large avocado, ripe
   2 celery stalks
   1/8 cup lemon juice, fresh
   2 garlic cloves
   1/2 bunch parsley
   1/2 cup basil and thyme, fresh
   1/3 tsp Celtic sea salt
   1 heaping tbsp nutritional yeast
   1 tbsp kelp powder
   2 cups fresh spring water
   4 tbsp of hemp seed nuts (or use your favorite nut milk)

Blend to desired consistency. (Always add water as needed)

Serves 2 to 4

Green Goddess Soup

Place in the blender in this order:

   2 medium tomatoes (chopped in large chunks)
   2 big handfuls of spinach (or 1 handful of spinach and 3 kale leaves unstemmed)
   2 or 3 celery stalks (chopped)
   1 or 2 cloves of garlic
   1/2 lemon (fresh-squeezed)
   1 1/2 avocados (peeled)
   1/4 tbsp sea salt
   1/2 cup of fresh basil

Cayenne pepper to taste

Blend to heavenly consistency....

Pour it into bowls and add some fresh thyme as an edible garnish.

This soup is cool, creamy, and unbelievably good! You can also try adding some cucumber or red pepper, or whatever herbs you're into.

Go anyway you want with this...and enjoy the Goddess!

Serves 2

Curry Soup

1 small organic cauliflower, cut into florets
1 red pepper, cored and deseeded
1 ripe avocado
2 garlic cloves, peeled
1/4 cup sweet onion, chopped
1/4 cup fresh squeezed lemon juice
2 heaping tbsp raw sesame tahini
2 tbsp brown rice miso (or another kind)
1 tbsp turmeric
1/2 to 1 tbsp of curry powder (depending on how spicy you like it)
1 tbsp Braggs Liquid Aminos
2 cups Almond Mylk (adding more to reach desired consistency)

You can optionally use spring water in this recipe in place of the almond mylk and add in a couple tbsp of olive oil to balance things out.

This is one of my personal favorites!

Serves 2

Sweet Broccoli Soup

- 4 cups chopped broccoli
- 1 avocado
- 2 cloves of garlic
- 1 big tbsp of red onion
- 2 tbsp of raw honey
- 1 tbsp of olive oil
- 1/2 tsp of cumin
- 1 tsp of sea salt
- 1/8 tsp of turmeric
- 1/8 tsp of black pepper
- 3 cups of almond mylk

Blend to desired consistency.

Serves 2

Home-style Green Tomato Soup (Juicer Style)

- 4 medium tomatoes
- 2 broccoli stalks
- 1 large carrot
- 1 handful of leafy greens (kale, spinach, romaine, etc.)
- 2 cloves of garlic
- 2 ribs of celery

Run all of these veggies through your juicer then put them into a warm pot with some freshly sautéed onions (use a couple tbsp of the juice to sauté the onions), add cayenne pepper, sea salt, and organic garlic powder to taste. Be sure to only warm the soup to retain all of the vital nutrients and enzymes that are lost in cooking. (A good test is being able to put your finger in it comfortably.) Pour into a bowl or thermos (I like to use a thermos) and sprinkle in some dulse flakes for extra nutritional power.

This soup is a bit greener than the classic canned imposter, but it sure is *good!*

Serves 2

DRESSINGS

Creamy Italian Dressing
 1 cup extra virgin olive oil
 1 1/2 cups fresh basil
 2 cups fresh parsley (approx. ? bunch)
 1/3 cup dried Italian Seasoning (Mixture of thyme, oregano, basil, etc.)
 1 tbsp red onion
 2 garlic cloves
 1 large lemon fresh-squeezed
 1 1/2 tbsp raw honey
 1 tsp Celtic sea salt

Blend all ingredients in your blender. Chill at least 30 minutes before serving. The longer it sits, the more the flavors get to mingle, and the results are beyond words!

Suggested serving with a big bowl of fresh salad greens, tomato, diced avocado, radishes (cut into match sticks), your favorite sprouts, and sprinkle dulse flakes over the top for a truly beautiful salad.

Yields approx. 3 cups. Keeps 2 to 3 days in the refrigerator.

5-Star French Dressing

1 cup fresh carrot juice
1/2 avocado
1 garlic clove, peeled
2 tbsp fresh-squeezed lemon juice
1/2 cup fresh parley (chopped), or 2 tbsp fresh dill
1/4 tbsp paprika
1/4 tsp Celtic sea salt

Prepare the carrot juice with a juicer. Transfer the carrot juice to your blender, along with the rest of the ingredients and blend to a creamy consistency.

Yields approx. 1 1/2 cups. Keeps 1 day.

Golden Greek Dressing

(A bit like Honey Mustard but with more of a kick!)

1 cup of olive oil
2 cloves of garlic
1/4 cup of diced red onion
3/4 tsp of sea salt
1/4 tsp of black pepper
1 big handful of fresh basil
2 tbsp of dried oregano
1 tbsp of ground mustard seed (most important ingredient)
3/4 cup of Apple Cider Vinegar (Braggs brand is the best ever!)

Add all ingredients to the blender and blend until smooth.

Blender Chef Tip: Add half of the olive oil and Apple Cider Vinegar with all of the other ingredients, blend until smooth, add the rest and then blend again.

This dressing serves 4 people heartily with a large salad.

Salad recommendation:
- Spinach and Baby Lettuces
- Radishes (matchstick style/sliced thin) or use shredded carrots (radishes are one of the best sources of organic sulfur, which is a beauty mineral)
- Diced tomato
- Avocado cubed (or some raw Greek olives)
- Kelp granules
- Maybe toss on some dehydrated pumpkin seeds, pistachios, or hemp seeds and enjoy!

Yields approx. 1 1/2 cups. Keeps 3 to 5 days in the refrigerator.

Easy Caesar

2 large tbsp of spicy mustard
1/2 fresh squeezed lemon
2 tbsp of hemp oil or olive oil
Pinch of sea salt
Dash of black pepper
Dash of garlic powder

Mix all ingredients together in a bowl, and you have fresh Caesar dressing.

Or to make a bigger batch put your ingredients in a blender (the magic bullet short cup is excellent here) using 1 or 2 garlic cloves instead of the garlic powder and basically double or triple the other ingredients.

The Classic

    1/2 cup of Olive oil
    1/4 cup Noma Shoyu (or Braggs Liquid Aminos)
    1/2 cup of Apple Cider Vinegar
    1/4 cup of lemon juice
    2 garlic cloves (shredded)

You can simply pour all of the ingredients into a bottle and shake it up.

Yields approx. 1 1/2 cups. Keeps 3 to 5 days in the refrigerator.

Honey Vinaigrette

    1/2 cup of apple cider vinegar
    1/4 cup of olive oil
    1/4 cup of lemon juice
    3 tbsp of raw honey
    1/2 tsp of Celtic sea salt

Blend all ingredients in your blender.

Yields approx. 1 1/2 cups. Keeps 3 to 5 days in the refrigerator.

Asante Sana Dressing

- 1/4 cup of olive oil
- 2 garlic cloves
- 2 tbsp of red onion
- 2 dates soaked
- 1 tbsp fresh ginger chopped
- 1 tbsp of raw honey
- 1 cup of raw almond butter
- 1 tbsp of Noma Shoyu or Braggs Liquid Aminos
- 1/4 tsp of cayenne pepper
- 1 lemon, juiced

Water added as needed to reach desired consistency (We like it pretty thick)

Blend all ingredients in a blender until smooth.

Yields approx. 2 cups. Keeps 2 to 3 days in the refrigerator.

This dressing literally transformed my life.
Thank you, Mama Mukami.

Recipes

80/20 Raw Options

These meals are some "transitional" live food options that are easy, mostly raw/living, and give you some options for when you're on the go. These are also nice for introducing other people into great nutrition, great living, and experiencing for themselves that these foods are tasty, satisfying and fun to eat.

Creamy Red Pepper Wrap

Place your wrap on a plate (Ezekiel brand is the best) and spread a generous amount of Hummus lengthwise and just off-center on your wrap Next add all of your fresh veggies (we like shredded carrot, tomato, lettuce, avocado, dulse and maybe some mushrooms or olives). Wrap it up, then pack it up or eat it up! Have with a fresh side salad and enjoy!

Promise Sandwich

Lightly toast two slices of sprouted grain bread. Place the toast on a plate and add a generous amount of avocado to each slice. Next add fresh lettuce, sliced tomato, and clover spouts to one slice. Add fresh basil leaves, cayenne pepper, and a little garlic powder to the other slice. Place one half on top of the other half, cut your sandwich diagonally. Serve with a medium salad and enjoy your new favorite lunch!

Easy Pita Pizzas

Place a whole grain pita on a plate and cut it into four pieces. After that, spread a generous layer of hummus over the entire pita (Matter of Flax makes a good hummus option). Add shredded lettuce, diced avocado, diced tomato, and grilled portabella mushrooms and/or olives on top. This is an incredible pizza experience, and it's super easy!

Note: It is tremendously beneficial to have either a fresh salad or fresh vegetable juice when you have any meal of cooked food. This is because of the vast enzymatic benefits and the vital aid in digestion of the cooked foods. But above all, enjoy your food, enjoy your experiences, and be truly grateful that you are giving your body the nourishment that it deserves.

A Note on Enzyme Inhibitors

Although nuts, seeds, beans, and other legumes have numerous health benefits, basically all of them have what are known as *enzyme inhibitors* enveloping them by nature. These inhibitors sometimes make it more difficult for you to digest these foods. This is why some people say that beans give them gas, or eating more than a few nuts upsets their stomach. This is due to the enzyme inhibitors not being dissolved. Either they have eaten beans from a can, or the beans or nuts that they've eaten were not properly prepared. All that needs to be done is to simply *soak them for the appropriate amount of time.* To actually activate the enzymes in them (thus unlocking all of the remarkable health benefits) they have to be soaked for the corresponding time from the table below so that the enzyme inhibitors are dissolved. Additionally, some beans, seeds, and grains can actually sprout, which massively increases their nutritional value.

	Soaking Time	**Sprouting Time**
Almonds	8 hours	N/A
Walnuts	4 hours	N/A
Sunflower Seeds	4 hours	1-2 days
Flax Seeds	1 hour	N/A
Barley & Wild Rice	9 hours	3-5 days
Wheat Berries	8 hours	2-3 days
Lentil Beans	8 hours	3 days
All Other Beans	Approximately 6 hours	
All Other Nuts	Approximately 6 hours	

FRESH JUICE RECIPES

Anytime is a good time for a revitalizing fresh-made juice, Try one of these for breakfast or anytime!

Super Anti-Aging Drink
8 medium carrots
1/2 bunch of parsley
3 large handfuls of spinach

Skin-Glow Beauty Drink
1 apple
1 cucumber (skin intact. Be sure it's organic!)
4 ribs of celery

Body Builder
5 or 6 kale leaves (dinosaur kale is a good choice)
4 ribs of celery
1 or 2 green Granny Smith apples
1/2 lemon peeled (with white pith remaining intact)

Energizer Bunny
5 medium carrots
5 ribs of celery

Sweetie Green
2 apples
2 carrots
2 ribs of celery
1 tbsp of Ormus Greens (or another Green SuperFood powder: Spirulina Sun Is Shining SuperFood, Vitamineral Green, etc.)

Lion Juice
2 big handfuls of dandelion greens
4 ribs of celery
1 sweet red apple

Life-Force Juice
4 carrots (tailed and topped)
3 big handfuls of clover sprouts
1 red apple

Pure Rejuvenation
1 cucumber (skin intact)
1 apple
3 handfuls of spinach (or kale)
1/2 lemon, peeled (with white pith remaining intact)

Sweet Beet
1 apple
2 carrots
4 celery stalks
1 beet

Fountain of Youth
1 cucumber (skin intact)
1 handful of dandelion greens
1 or 2 sweet red apples

ACC
2 apples
2 carrots
2 celery stalks

Green Monster
2 green apples
2 kiwis
handful of green grapes (seeded is best)
1 tbsp of Ormus Greens (or another green powder)

Tropical Tango
2 oranges
2 mangos
1 kiwi
1 apple

Zesty Orange-Carrot
3 oranges
1 carrot
1 1/2-inch piece of fresh ginger root

Recipes

Watermelon Thirst Quencher

Take plenty of juicy pieces of seeded watermelon and run them through your juicer. This one is magic!

Juicing Tips:

- Whenever juicing leafy greens (spinach, kale, dandelion, etc.), be sure to ball them up tightly in your hand before putting them into the juicer. Always follow the greens with a juicier vegetable or fruit (a cucumber, rib of celery, etc.) to push any remaining juice through.
- Alternate the different vegetables/fruits while you are putting them through the juicer.

  Example: To make the *Pure Rejuvenation Drink,* put through the juicer in the following order:

  Apple slices, 1/2 cucumber, handful of spinach (tightly squeezed into a ball), peeled lemon, 1/2 cucumber.

- When pressing leafy greens through the juicer, use the press and release method to enable your juicer to stay running and to extract the greatest amount of juice from your greens.

  Simple method: Press the greens down with the food guider, then quickly release. Continue to guide the greens through at this steady press and release rhythm until they are completely through the extractor. And, as always, follow the greens with a higher water content vegetable or fruit.

  Always choose organic foods whenever possible.

Good Food on the Go!
And Super Treats for Everyone!

SuperFood Trail Mix
Goji berries
Cacao nibs
Raw cashews

Raw SuperFood Mountain Mix
Cacao nibs
Mulberries
Sunflower seeds
Almonds
Pumpkin seeds

Magic Mix
Cacao nibs
Mulberries
Coconut flakes
Raw cashews

World Traveler's Mix
Dried cranberries
Pumpkin seeds
Raw cashews
Hunza raisins
Goji berries

Recipes

Cashew Butter Planets

2 cups of raw cashew butter

2 tbsp of soaked flax seeds (soaked at least 1 hour. Overnight is good.)

2 tbsp of hemp seed nuts

2 tbsp of raw honey

1/4 tsp of sea salt.

1 ripe banana diced (optional)

Combine all of the ingredients into a large bowl and mix it all together. Then grab enough of the mixture in your hand to make a golf ball-sized sphere. As you finish rolling each one, place them in a freezer-safe container lined with parchment paper. Give each planet its own little space. After you finish one layer, lay parchment paper on top and create another layer. Continue this process until all of the mixture is used. (Be sure to clean your fingers off the old-fashioned way when you're done!) Put a tight-fitting top on the container and place it in the freezer to become something special!

These are great for a quick snack after a workout or if you're walking out the door and you need a quick energy boost. Kids love these too! They are especially good when you let them thaw out for just a couple of minutes before you enjoy them, or simply eat them straight out of the freezer like ice cream! How's that? Ice cream with massive health benefits, taste incredible, and no guilt! That's right, let go of the guilt...put it down...let it go... *You're now eating the best food on the planet!*

GRRRAW-NOLA

Sprouted sunflower seeds

Cacao nibs

Goji berries

Hemp seed nuts

Chopped walnuts (and/or chopped almonds. I like to "Honey" these, meaning I mix them in some raw honey)

Serve in a bowl with a diced banana, cinnamon and your favorite nut milk.

ICE CREAM *(That's Right!)*

Special Note: This one is going to flip you out!

One instruction: Take some frozen bananas out of the freezer (about 3 is good) and put them in the food processor. When you see what happens when they are spinning around becoming this amazing, silky, creamy goodness... It is an experience everyone should have. Eat it as is, or add your favorite toppings:

Cacao nibs
Chopped pecans
Goji berries
Hemp nuts
Bee Pollen
Fresh strawberries or homemade strawberry sauce

Extra Tip: Add Cacao powder, Mesquite, Maca, and a pinch of sea salt to the food processor with the ice cream and... You can imagine!

CHOCOLATE-COVERED STRAWBERRY PUDDING

1 1/2 cups of frozen strawberries
2 tbsp of cacao powder
1 tbsp of Maca
1 ripe avocado
2 tbsp of raw honey
Coconut water (added as needed to reach desired consistency)

Blend all ingredients in a blender and watch the magic happen.

You have to taste this to believe it... It is crazy good!
This one could have easily been in the SuperFood Smoothie/Drink section.

You simply add more coconut water and it will take on a more smoothie-like consistency. You can optionally use frozen blueberries for another amazing version. Just add a bit of cinnamon or mesquite to the mix and you've got a creamy, rich blueberry-chocolate shake.

DINO-FIGS
Dried Calimyrna or Turkish figs
Almond butter (or Cashew butter)
Cinnamon

Slice the figs open, stuff them with almond butter and sprinkle with cinnamon.

GO NUTS!
For great energy and performance have a couple of big handfuls of your favorite seasoned and dehydrated raw nuts or seeds (Ex., Tamari Almonds, Pesto Walnuts, Buttery Pumpkin seeds with Celtic Sea Salt, Brazil Nuts, Sweet and Spicy Chipotle Pistachios, Creamy Macadamias, etc.)

Superfood Bars
"Wild Bar" *Mountain Mint* or *Mayan Spice*
"Active Greens" and others by *Organic Food Bar*
"Cinnamon Raisin" and others by *Raw Organic Food Bar*
Prana Bars, Vega, and *RawVolution* has some good options too.

Note: By far, the best snack food that you can treat yourself to is fresh *organic* fruit! If you need to have something that you can keep with you in your book bag, in your purse, or in your office drawer, the best thing you can get your hands on are wildcrafted or organic Goji berries or Inca Berries. These incredible berries are quick and easy, and not to mention loaded with nutrition!

THE BEST BONUS NOTE EVER

All meal options are absolutely 100% interchangeable. If you want to have an amazing SuperFood Smoothie for dinner, then do it! If you want to have The GUAC and flax crackers for lunch, then do that! Mix it up, because when you're eating truly nourishing food, you don't have to go by the rest of the world's standards. They'll catch on eventually… For now, just continue to focus on *your* health and do what works best for you! On occasion, my wife and I have had the Raw Ice Cream and some other raw treats for dinner and it was absolutely incredible!

It is such a freeing experience when you let go of all the labels and the illusionary restrictions that have been keeping us in bondage for so long. It's not about any of that stuff. It is about reconnecting to what is real and most important about us, and that is our true nature of *Oneness*.

What is presented to you here is merely a taste of the endless meal ideas that can be created by you and your family. With the increase in your consciousness, so too comes an exponential increase in your creativity. It is simply a matter of attuning yourself to that higher frequency. When you start to eat the good stuff, then all of the bad stuff will naturally push itself out of the picture. With the power of right thinking and right nutrition, this is when you can't help but to carry a higher frequency. This is when you will truly realize, understand, and experience *The Best Health Ever!*

BONUS 1:
5 Essentials for Achieving Remarkable Physical Fitness

#1 Cleanse and Detoxify Your Body

In all matters of longevity and rejuvenation, there is no greater method than through cleansing and detoxification of the body. A structured cleansing program allows for your body to essentially rid itself of all of the "stuff" that's not *you*. On a cellular level, when your body is overrun with toxic residues, heavy metals, excess mucus, environmental waste products, and debris from undigested food, then obviously your system isn't going to be running at its optimum level. Your cells, blood, tissues, organs, muscles, etc., are going to be more difficult to change when there is so much debris in the way blocking the inherent flow; or on a visual level, the translation of your desired goals into your realized physical health.

When your cells are clean and clear, there is an unquestionable feeling of vitality in the body. That increase in the energy flow results in a heightened state of clarity, the elimination of excess fat, an increase in the production of "good" hormones like HGH, reduction or elimination of disease from the body, and an overall feeling of well-being. For more information on Cleansing and Detoxification, check out my book, *The Detox Success System*.

#2 Participate in an Exercise Program That You Enjoy

Life *is* exercise. The only thing is that most of us have subjected ourselves to a very sedentary lifestyle. So we are required to attain our physical fitness through different exercise programs to give our bodies the movement that they were designed to have. This doesn't mean that it has to be rigid, or that it has to be a struggle. This doesn't mean that you can't have an absolutely amazing time doing it! The only trouble is that most people have mentally connected a great deal of pain to working out and exercising. But they are completely unaware of it because it is lodged in the subconscious mind.

This is why people will know that they "should" workout, or they "should" participate in an exercise program but they just don't, and end up giving every excuse in the book as to why they're not doing it. The truth is that if it were really enjoyable to them, if it provided them with an intense amount of *pleasure,* then they would be there doing their desired exercise program and feeling great. *No matter what!* As a matter of fact, it would be so enjoyable to them that it would simply become a part of who they are. And denying themselves the pleasure that they receive from their exercise would be like denying themselves of good food, drink, and excellent companionship. It would truly be a vital piece missing from their life. The key is to reprogram those limiting beliefs that it has to be hard, and it has to be a struggle, and begin associating intense pleasure with the exercise program that you enjoy.

So here's a powerful piece of information for Fat Loss and Physical Fitness:

It's all about getting your body in a high metabolic state. Muscle is the body's fat burning "machinery." The more muscle you have, the more fat you burn. It's as simple as that. I'm not talking about you carrying around some huge amount of muscle to see significant fat loss. I'm talking about simply increasing the amount of lean muscle that you have right now and *instantly* getting an upgrade in your metabolism. You will then be burning fat at a higher rate just doing your normal day-to-day activities. Now how easy is that?! It's simply because you have equipped yourself with more fat-burning machinery. For more on Fat Loss and some of the Best Workout Programs on the planet, pick up *The Fat Loss Code* at www.TheShawnStevensonModel.com

#3 Get a Good PROBIOTIC

Probiotic literally translates as "Pro" meaning *for* and "biotic" meaning *life*. So probiotic literally means *for life!* Guess what Anti-biotic means? That's right; "anti" means *Against* and "biotic" is *Life*. Antibiotic *literally means* against life! Guess which one you've had? Now we're putting some powerful realizations together. You have more bacteria in your body than you even have human cells. That's how it is supposed to be. Now the only question is which team is controlling the game; is it the good guys (the friendly Flora, beneficial bacteria) or is it the bad guys (the bad bacteria, lower-level funguses, yeast, Candida, etc.)? The friendly flora create the majority of your immune system weapons, they create vitamins and minerals for you, and they also aid in the digestion and assimilation of the food that you eat. If you can't digest your food properly, then everything that you eat will be injurious to you and causing an immune system response. Get the winning team in the game.

#4 Take MSM and Camu Camu

One of the main nutrients that you are made of is sulfur. It is truly one of the key elements of *life*. It's critical in the regeneration and support of healthy muscles, ligaments, and tissues; as well as for regenerating and expressing healthy skin, hair, and nails. Sulfur is truly a beauty mineral.

MSM (MethylSulfonylMethane) is an Organic Sulfur Compound that is found in all living organisms. When your body lacks adequate amounts of MSM the cells become rigid and "dry." This is a strong determinant of the aging process.

When your body has the proper supply of sulfur in your tissues, this allows for the regeneration of new, healthy tissues. It only makes sense that if your body doesn't have what it needs to keep you young and vibrant, then obviously it would start to break down at accelerated rates. Have you had your MSM today?

Essentials for Achieving Remarkable Physical Fitness

MSM is one of the most remarkable substances that I have ever seen, point blank. I have seen it have the most remarkable effects on more people (including myself) than any other "supplement" out there. But here's the thing, it's really not a simple "supplement" so to speak. When you are getting it from a plant-derived source, then it's an organic sulfur compound that is derived in the rain process and (again) *it is one of the main things that you're made of!* It's important to continue to up-level the amount of MSM that you take over the weeks and months to notice some really powerful benefits. Now you know, so take action to add it in.

MSM works in conjunction with Vitamin C to build new tissues. Vitamin C helps support collagen production and increases longevity in many different ways. In the field of nutrition we've found that the most powerful source of Vitamin C are Botanical Vitamin C sources, rather than synthetic Vitamin C sources. The highest and most potent source of Vitamin C in the world (by far) is the Camu Camu Berry. In a comparative study of the most powerful botanicals in the world Camu Camu ranks #1 in effectiveness for:

Asthma
Atherosclerosis
Cataracts
Colds
Edema
Gingivitis/Periodontal disease
Glaucoma
Hepatitis
Infertility
Migraine headaches
Osteoarthritis
Painkiller
Parkinson's disease
(And this is just some of the list)

Yes, this is a truly remarkable botanical. And people are really waking up to this. You can get this as a raw, dehydrated powder and simply add it to your water, juice, smoothies, etc. Just add a little bit in and get all the benefits.

Understand you always want to get the absolute best products that are available to you. Why get the second best? I set the intention, opened myself up to receive the best products available, and they showed up for me. These are truly the absolute best products in the world that I am sharing with you. Made by the best companies, with the most integrity, and they have put the most care and consideration into their products. Visit www.TheShawnStevensonModel.com.

#5 Chew Your Food!

Upwards of 80% of the energy most people use every day is spent on digesting the food that they're eating. This leaves only about 20% of the energy for doing everything else they may want to do like: thinking, walking, talking, working, creating abundance, **_getting in shape!_** Give your body and your life a simple gift that can pay-off big dividends: chew your food thoroughly so that your body doesn't have to spend so much energy breaking down big pieces of grub that are going down into your stomach. Your food should be in liquid form *before* you swallow it. Plus, the best thing ever you could do is to eat at least one blended or juiced meal per day like: a delicious Superfood Shake, a Fresh Blended Soup, or a Fresh-Made Alkaline Juice.

One of the most powerful things that you can do to increase your health *instantly* is to bring complete awareness to your food when you are eating. If you are not in the habit of taking time with your food and truly appreciating what you are doing, then chances are you are tossing more food into your body than you are even aware of. And it doesn't matter if it's a bag of processed cookies made by those elves, or a bag of raw organic flax crackers; if you are not bringing awareness to what you are doing, you may look up and see that the bag is empty and your stomach has more stuff in it then you intended.

A wise, old saying goes like this:

> *"Chew your juice and Drink your food."*

Bonus 2:
Menu for Weight Loss (Monday)

The #1 practice in the nutritional regimen of anyone who is seeking extraordinary health and vitality is the consumption of fresh, clean water.

Upon rising:

1 liter of Fresh, Clean Water
MSM (1 to 3 tbsp)
Camu Camu Berry Powder (1/2 tbsp)
Pinch of Celtic Sea Salt
Fresh squeezed lemon juice (optional)

Add all of these powerful cleansing and rebuilding nutrients to a bottle with a lid; shake it up and have your inner bath.

This will help to flush your system out and transition your body for breaking your overnight fast. After using the restroom, proceed to having your breakfast. (Be sure it is at least 30 minutes later.)

Breakfast:

The Maca Shake (aka The Fat Loss Express!)

Lunch:

Skin-Glow Beauty Salad

Afternoon Snack:

Have your choice of fresh fruit

Dinner:

Easy Nori Rolls + A Small Green Salad + Supplemental Enzymes

Evening:

Have 2 tbsp of Apple Cider Vinegar with 1 oz. of spring water.

Drink water throughout the day! The only recommendation here is to wait at least 30 minutes after drinking water before having a meal and to wait at least one hour after a meal before drinking water. This is to ensure proper digestion of your food.

Menu for Weight Loss
(Tuesday)

Upon rising:

1 liter of Fresh, Clean Water
MSM
Camu Camu Berry Powder
Pinch of Celtic Sea Salt
Fresh squeezed lemon juice (optional)

Breakfast:

The Chocolate Champion

Lunch:

Superhero Salad

Afternoon Tonic:

Skin-Glow Beauty Drink + 1 tsp of Blue-Green Algae

Dinner:

Creamy Broccoli Soup
(Make enough for tomorrow's lunch too. This is good!)

Drink water throughout the day! The only recommendation here is to wait at least 30 minutes after drinking water before having a meal and to wait at least one hour after a meal before drinking water. This is to ensure proper digestion of your food.

Menu for Weight Loss (Wednesday)

Upon rising:
1 liter of Fresh, Clean Water
MSM
Camu Camu Berry Powder
Pinch of Celtic Sea Salt
Fresh squeezed lemon juice (optional)

Breakfast:
Ultimate Longevity Elixir

Lunch:
Creamy Broccoli Soup

Afternoon Snack:
Have your choice of fresh fruit

Dinner:
Macho Tacos + Supplemental Enzymes

Evening:
Have 2 tbsp of Apple Cider Vinegar with 1 oz. of spring water.

Drink water throughout the day! The only recommendation here is to wait at least 30 minutes after drinking water before having a meal and to wait at least one hour after a meal before drinking water. This is to ensure proper digestion of your food.

Menu for Weight Loss
(Thursday)

Upon rising:
1 liter of Fresh, Clean Water
MSM
Camu Camu Berry Powder
Pinch of Celtic Sea Salt
Fresh squeezed lemon juice (optional)

Breakfast:
Ultimate Longevity Elixir

Lunch:
Super Salad + Beauty Enzymes

Afternoon Tonic:
Skin-Glow Beauty Drink + 1 tsp to 1 tbsp of Blue-Green Algae

Dinner:
Seventh Heaven Soup + Supplemental Enzymes

Evening:
Have 2 tbsp of Apple Cider Vinegar with 1 oz. of spring water.

Drink water throughout the day! The only recommendation here is to wait at least 30 minutes after drinking water before having a meal and to wait at least one hour after a meal before drinking water. This is to ensure proper digestion of your food.

Menu for Weight Loss
(Friday)

Upon rising:
1 liter of Fresh, Clean Water
MSM
Camu Camu Berry Powder
Pinch of Celtic Sea Salt
Fresh squeezed lemon juice (optional)

Breakfast:
Have any of the shakes or juices from the recipe section, or come up with your own "Specialty" drink.

Lunch:
Cado & Cracker Mini-Sandwiches + Supplemental Enzymes

Afternoon Tonic:
Skin-Glow Beauty Drink + 1 tsp of Blue-Green Algae

Dinner:
Fresh Green Salad with avocado, tomato, radishes, broccoli sprouts Italian Dressing. Sprinkle dulse flakes on top + Supplemental Enzymes.

Evening/ Dessert:
Have a couple of Cashew Butter Planets.

Drink water throughout the day! The only recommendation here is to wait at least 30 minutes after drinking water before having a meal and to wait at least one hour after a meal before drinking water. This is to ensure proper digestion of your food.

Menu for Weight Loss
(Saturday)

Upon rising:

1 liter of Fresh, Clean Water
MSM
Camu Camu Berry Powder
Pinch of Celtic Sea Salt
Fresh squeezed lemon juice (optional)

Breakfast:

SUPERMAN or WONDER WOMAN Drink

Lunch:

Chocolate Dream

Afternoon Tonic:

Body Builder

Dinner:

Have your choice of any of the recipes or any Raw/Live Food recipe that you're into + Supplemental Enzymes.

Drink water throughout the day! The only recommendation here is to wait at least 30 minutes after drinking water before having a meal and to wait at least one hour after a meal before drinking water. This is to ensure proper digestion of your food.

Menu for Weight Loss
(Sunday)

Upon rising:

1 liter of Fresh, Clean Water
MSM
Camu Camu Berry Powder
Pinch of Celtic Sea Salt
Fresh squeezed lemon juice (optional)

Breakfast:

Today you will be giving your body some extra time for detoxification. Have 2 tbsp of Apple Cider Vinegar with 2 oz. of spring water. Afterwards take some time and do a little reading on some great things that pertain to your health and vitality, Success Technology, or do some journaling. Or simply just take out some time and do some meditation or quite reflection to assist your body in the detoxification process.

Lunch:

Have a fresh fruit salad that includes papaya, kiwi, strawberries, blackberries, and 1 banana.

Afternoon Tonic:

Super Anti-aging Drink or Body Builder

Dinner:

Fresh Green Salad with avocado, tomato, carrots, kelp granules, dehydrated pumpkin seeds and Golden Greek Dressing

---

Drink water throughout the day!

Additional Tips for Weight Loss:

Tip 1: It is important to understand how the body actually got into the state of carrying excess weight in the first place. The vast majority of the situation is a case in which the cells of the body have become inflamed due to the consumption of inflammatory, acidic foods. When you consume lifeless/ denatured foods, in an effort to keep your major organs protected, your body will simply respond by shoving the toxic residues into your fat cells. As you continue to eat this way, over time, one may think that they are "picking up weight," but what is actually happening is your body is in a state of chronic inflammation.

The top three inflammatory foods are:

1. **Pasteurized dairy products.**

    This is the #1 mucous-forming food and it actually causes an instant histamine reaction when consumed. Visit NotMilk.com to help heal yourself and your family of allergies, asthma, obesity-related illnesses and find out how to avoid the harmful effects that pasteurized dairy has on your body.

2. **Cooked Grains (Especially cooked wheat)**

    The protein that is in high concentration in wheat, known as Gluten, is incredibly inflammatory when it is cooked. It causes your body and even your face to become puffy and bloated. You will notice more and more that there are "Gluten-free" products on the store shelves. But it is not the Gluten that is harming people and causing allergic reactions; it is cooking a grain that isn't intended to be cooked. Many of the storied armies of the world were "grain-feed" armies; like the Romans, the Greeks, etc. We all know the great physical culture that they exuded. We still admire their beauty and aesthetics today. The difference is they didn't destroy the grain first and then eat it. They ate it in its natural state.

By soaking, sprouting, marinating, and combining it with other delicious raw foods, it can truly be made into some amazing culinary delights. It can be a very potent strength building energy source.

3. **Processed sugar**

You can write a whole book on this one alone. Cooked sugar is a drug. It tears up the body up in ways that are completely horrific. When you consume a natural sugar, it is used as an energy source or stored in your cells as fat for possible use as energy later. This is with *all* sugars. Cooked sugar is completely denatured, so your body doesn't recognize it as a natural sugar and when it is consumed it literally short-wires your metabolism, devastates your pancreas function, and because you don't have the aliesthetic taste change that you get with a natural sugar (which is basically a shut-off valve), you can take in massive amounts of this stuff and it's literally rampaging around in your blood stream tearing up whatever it can and causing disease, illnesses, and obesity to manifest seemingly out of nowhere. Once you see this for yourself, and the effect that it has on the people around you, it is bordering on madness to even mess around with this stuff.

People seem to blind themselves to what they see sugar as being (which is an engraved societal conditioning). So to specify what we're talking about, here it is:
- All sugar from the store shelves
- High-Fructose corn syrup and other processed sweeteners
- Soda of any and all kinds (It actually burns going down!)
- Pasteurized fruit juices (This is *all* of the juices on the store shelves.) When you make a fresh juice it oxidizes very quickly. That's why all of the juices on the store shelves are pasteurized (cooked) so that they can sit on the store shelves for weeks and even months on end. Once you cook it, you kill all of the life-

giving nutrition that was once in it, and you are left drinking pure processed sugar. Let me say that again: *You are left drinking pure, processed sugar.* Nothing else.

- Cooked starches (i.e. wheat, rice, pasta), and this does include "Whole Wheat Pasta," "Whole Wheat Bagels" and there's even sugary "Whole Wheat kids cereals" that are being sold as a better option for you. Please understand, it's all sly marketing. Shift your attention to the *absolute abundance* that you have available to you now. Most people eat the same 12 to 15 foods every single day (different forms of the same foods), when there are over 50,000 different types of food that you can be enjoying. So don't limit yourself and allow your decisions to be made for you. Take your power back and put your intention on pleasurable abundance, and it will show up for you.

To remedy the situation of having a body that is "overweight" (which is really a state of over-acidity and chronic inflammation), you simply need to eat anti-inflammatory foods, and of course, eliminate the cause of the inflammation. Just observe as the weight, and all of the stuff that's not you, falls away. When I refer to anti-inflammatory foods, I am referring to foods that are predominantly alkaline forming, juicy, and highly mineralized. Many of these foods and recipes have been presented to you in this book. For more, visit www.TheShawnStevensonModel.com.

Tip 2: Begin a probiotic regimen along with your morning water as needed for your particular state of health. This is to replenish and create the proper environment in your body for health, fitness, and the desired weight to be achieved.

Tip 3: Take Supplemental Enzymes to help you assimilate your food and clear up the debris and waste products that are inhibiting the flow in your system.

Tip 4: Complete a structured cleanse and detox program. Check out The Detox Success System at www.TheShawnStevensonModel.com

Tip 5: Participate in a regular exercise program that *you* enjoy!
It's for you and no one else. Have fun and give your body (who is your ultimate companion) what it really deserves; Freedom of Movement, Adventure, and Fun. Get out there and *live!*

Bonus 3:
Menu for Increasing Muscle Mass (Monday)

NOTE: This regimen is to be combined with a regular resistance training program to facilitate the increased nutritional intake as described here in this menu. The #1 practice in the nutritional regimen of anyone who is seeking extraordinary health and vitality is the consumption of fresh, clean water.

Muscle is 70% water, 22% protein, and 7 to 8% lipids or fat.

Upon rising:

1 liter of Fresh, Clean Water
MSM (1 to 3 tbsp)
Camu Camu Berry Powder (1/2 tbsp)
Pinch of Celtic Sea Salt
Fresh squeezed lemon juice (optional)

Add all of these powerful cleansing and rebuilding nutrients to a bottle with a lid; shake it up and have your inner bath. This will help to flush your system out and transition your body for *breaking* your overnight *fast*. After using the restroom, proceed to having your breakfast. (Be sure it is at least 30 min. later)

Breakfast:

Noble Warrior Protein Drink + 1 Extra tbsp of flax oil

Lunch:

Ultimate Longevity Elixir + 1 or 2 extra tbsp of Hemp seeds

Afternoon Tonic:

32 oz. Pure Rejuvenation **Note:** It is very important to keep your body Alkaline. Having a fresh vegetable-based juice implemented in your training regimen will assist you in flushing out excess toxins, acids, and waste products that can accumulate in the body from exercise.

Dinner:

Superhero Salad + 2 Extra Tbsp of Pumpkin Seeds and 2 Extra tbsp of Olive oil in the dressing.

Drink water throughout the day! The only recommendation here is to wait at least 30 minutes after drinking water before having a meal and to wait at least one hour after a meal before drinking water. This is to ensure proper digestion of your food.

Menu for Increasing Muscle Mass
(Tuesday)

Upon rising:
1 liter of Fresh, Clean Water
MSM
Camu Camu Berry Powder
Pinch of Celtic Sea Salt
Fresh squeezed lemon juice (optional)

Breakfast:
Noble Warrior Protein Drink + 1 Extra tbsp of hemp oil

Lunch:
Large Bowl of Broccoli Soup + Supplemental Enzymes

Afternoon Snack:
Have 4 to 6 Dino-Figs

Dinner:
Large Fresh Green Salad with 2 avocados, tomato, carrots kelp granules, dehydrated pumpkin seeds and Golden Greek Dressing

---

Drink water throughout the day! The only recommendation here is to wait at least 30 minutes after drinking water before having a meal and to wait at least one hour after a meal before drinking water. This is to ensure proper digestion of your food.

Menu for Increasing Muscle Mass
(Wednesday)

Upon rising:

1 liter of Fresh, Clean Water
MSM
Camu Camu Berry Powder
Pinch of Celtic Sea Salt
Fresh squeezed lemon juice (optional)

Breakfast:

SUPERMAN or WONDER WOMAN DRINK

Lunch:

The Chocolate Champion + 2 Extra tbsp of hemp seeds

Afternoon:

Have 4 oz. of seasoned, dehydrated almonds, walnuts, or pistachios.

Dinner:

Large Fresh Green Salad with 2 avocados, tomato, carrots kelp granules, dehydrated pumpkin seeds and Golden Greek Dressing + Supplemental Enzymes

Evening:

(Optional) Have a few handfuls of Goji Berries, Inca Berries, or a Superfood Trail Mix

---

Drink water throughout the day! The only recommendation here is to wait at least 30 minutes after drinking water before having a meal and to wait at least one hour after a meal before drinking water. This is to ensure proper digestion of your food.

Menu for Increasing Muscle Mass
(Thursday)

Upon rising:
1 liter of Fresh, Clean Water
MSM
Camu Camu Berry Powder
Pinch of Celtic Sea Salt
Fresh squeezed lemon juice (optional)

Breakfast:
Flying High Smoothie

Lunch:
Large Bowl of Broccoli Soup + Supplemental Enzymes

Afternoon Tonic:
32 oz. Body Builder or Skin-Glow Beauty Drink

Dinner:
Nori Rules! (Load these up!)

Evening:
(Optional) Have a few handfuls of Goji Berries, Inca Berries, or a Superfood Trail Mix

---

Drink water throughout the day! The only recommendation here is to wait at least 30 minutes after drinking water before having a meal and to wait at least one hour after a meal before drinking water. This is to ensure proper digestion of your food.

Menu for Increasing Muscle Mass
(Friday)

Upon rising:
1 liter of Fresh, Clean Water
MSM
Camu Camu Berry Powder
Pinch of Celtic Sea Salt
Fresh squeezed lemon juice (optional)

Breakfast:
Chocolate Champion + 2 Extra tbsp of hemp seeds

Lunch:
Have any of the Superfood Elixirs from the recipe section, or come up with your own "Specialty" drink.

Afternoon Snack:
Have 4 oz. of seasoned, dehydrated almonds, walnuts, or pistachios.

Dinner:
Fresh Green Salad with 2 avocados, tomato, radishes, broccoli sprouts, and Italian Dressing + Sprinkle dulse flakes on top

Evening:
(Optional) Have some *Cashew Butter Planets*.

Drink water throughout the day! The only recommendation here is to wait at least 30 minutes after drinking water before having a meal and to wait at least one hour after a meal before drinking water. This is to ensure proper digestion of your food.

Menu for Increasing Muscle Mass
(Saturday)

Upon rising:

1 liter of Fresh, Clean Water
MSM
Camu Camu Berry Powder
Pinch of Celtic Sea Salt
Fresh squeezed lemon juice (optional)

Breakfast:

Flying High Smoothie

Lunch:

Curry Cauliflower Soup + drizzle 1 extra tbsp of olive oil over your soup after you pour it into your bowl.

Afternoon Tonic:

32 oz. Body Builder or Skin-Glow Beauty Drink

Dinner:

Macho Tacos. Or have your choice of any of the recipes, or any high Raw/Live Food recipe that you're into + Supplemental Enzymes.

Evening:

(Optional) Have a few handfuls of Goji Berries, Inca Berries, or a Superfood Trail Mix

---

Drink water throughout the day! The only recommendation here is to wait at least 30 minutes after drinking water before having a meal and to wait at least one hour after a meal before drinking water. This is to ensure proper digestion of your food.

Menu for Increasing Muscle Mass
(Sunday)

Upon rising:
1 liter of Fresh, Clean Water
MSM
Camu Camu Berry Powder
Pinch of Celtic Sea Salt
Fresh squeezed lemon juice (optional)

Breakfast:
Noble Warrior Protein Drink + 1 Extra tbsp of flax Oil

Lunch:
Large Bowl of Broccoli Soup + Supplemental Enzymes

Afternoon Snack:
Have a fresh fruit salad that includes papaya, kiwi, strawberries, blackberries, and 1 banana

Dinner:
Fresh Green Salad with 2 avocados, tomato, radishes, sprouts
Italian Dressing
+ Sprinkle dulse flakes on top
+ Supplemental Enzymes.

Drink water throughout the day! The only recommendation here is to wait at least 30 minutes after drinking water before having a meal and to wait at least one hour after a meal before drinking water. This is to ensure proper digestion of your food.

Additional Tips for Increasing Muscle Mass:

Tip 1: Once you are experienced in lifting, really shift your focus on muscle overload. This is basically driving the muscles beyond their normal threshold to maximize your gains in size and strength. After overloading the muscles during your workout, immediately switch your attention to proper rest and recovery. This is to facilitate the healing of your body so that you come back stronger and more muscularly developed each time. When you are lifting weights, you are actually tearing your muscle fibers, and breaking your body down in many aspects. Your "gains" are not really happening in the gym; all of the development actually happens afterward.

Here's a simple question to assist in understanding this better:
   Are you actually stronger at the *end* of your workout, after you've trained and worked your muscles intensely?

Of course not! The repairing process, as well as the proper healing and nutrition, allows for your body to come back stronger and more developed to surpass your previous physical capabilities. The real gains happen while you're sleeping. This is when your body releases the most Human Growth Hormone and other rejuvenating hormones and healing processes to give you the results that you worked for.

Tip 2: Align one of your meals (especially a Superfood Elixir) so that you can have it at the end of your workout session. Science has proven, time and time again, that if you want to make the greatest increases in your physical fitness, there is a powerful window of opportunity to fuel this advancement nutritionally. Having a powerful post-workout drink (preferably within 60 minutes after working out) is absolutely essential for this.

Tip 3: Begin a probiotic regimen along with your morning water and as needed for your particular state of health. This is to replenish and create the proper environment in your body for health, fitness, and the desired physique to be achieved.

Tip 4: Take Supplemental Enzymes to help you assimilate your food and clear up the debris and waste products that are inhibiting the flow in your system.

Tip 5: Participate in exercise programs that you enjoy doing. If you don't enjoy doing it, if it's not challenging and fun for you, then why are you even doing it? If you're not enjoying the process, then it's simply not going to last. It's all about having fun, discovering new and exciting challenges for you to accomplish, having a wide variety of workout programs to choose from, uncovering new and different ways of doing things, and enjoying the physical mastery that you attain. For cutting-edge workout information and some of the best exercise programs on the planet, visit www.TheShawnStevensonModel.com.

Bonus 4:
Prosperity of Beauty Foods

Foods Rich in Zinc

- Pumpkin seeds
- Macadamia nuts
- Pine nuts
- Cashews
- Coconuts
- Sunflower seeds
- Poppy seeds
- Sesame seeds
- Chayote
- Irish moss
- Spinach
- Wheat grass
- Alfalfa sprouts
- Radish sprouts
- Clover sprouts

Foods Rich in Iron

- Spinach
- Swiss chard
- Burdock root
- Cherries
- Cacao
- Sea vegetables
- Parley
- Wheatgrass and other grasses
- Cilantro
- Irish moss
- Kale
- Spirulina
- Asparagus
- Sauerkraut
- Mushrooms

Foods Rich in Sulfur

- Radishes
- Kale
- Mustard greens
- Broccoli
- Hot peppers
- Hemp nuts
- Garlic
- Onions
- Pumpkin seeds
- Arugula
- Watercress
- Aloe vera
- Spirulina
- Maca
- Beepollen

Foods Rich in Silicon

- Radishes
- Cucumber (in the skin)
- Romaine lettuce
- Alfalfa
- Bell peppers
- Tomatoes
- Nettles
- Oatstraw
- Horsetail
- Hemp leaves
- Onions
- Cabbage
- Oranges
- Almonds
- Oats (steel cut is best)

Foods Rich in Manganese

- Wild lettuces
- Arugula
- Hemp seeds
- Almonds
- Brazil nuts
- Cacao
- Spinach
- Kale
- Rasins
- Prunes
- Pineapples
- Pecans
- Watercress
- Sea vegetables (Dulse, kelp, etc.)
- Green tea

Foods Rich in Calcium

- Figs
- Blackberries
- Currants
- Kale
- Spinach
- Collards
- Almonds
- Brazil nuts
- Dandelion
- Parsley
- Mustard greens
- Sesame seeds
- Sunflower seeds
- Sea vegetables
- Carrots

Foods Rich in Magnesium

- Spinach
- Kale
- Swiss chard
- Cacao
- Almonds
- Hazelnuts
- Bananas
- Figs
- Okra
- Pumpkin seeds
- Sesame seeds
- Sunflower seeds
- Pine nuts
- Cashews
- Beet greens

Foods Rich in Vitamin C

- Camu Camu berries
- Citrus fruits (oranges, lemons)
- Bell peppers
- Broccoli
- Cauliflower
- Cantaloupe
- Kiwi
- Papaya
- Strawberries
- Acerola
- Cacao
- Goji berries
- Parseley
- Garlic
- Cabbage

Excellent Sources of EFA's

- Hemp seeds
- Hemp oil
- Flax seeds
- Flax oil
- Chia seeds
- Walnuts
- Macadamia nuts
- Olives
- Olive oil
- Borage oil
- Evening Primrose oil
- Marine Phytoplankton
- Coconuts
- Coconut oil
- Avocados

Excellent Sources of Probiotics and/or Prebiotics

- Sauerkraut
- Kim Chi
- Coconut Kefir
- Kombucha (growing your own is best)
- Rejuvelac (fermented drink made from grains; check the internet for recipes)
- Nut and Seed Cheeses
- Miso
- Noma Shoyu
- Tamari
- Raw Honey (especially Manuka)
- Yacon Root Syrup
- Berries (especially Goji berries)
- Wild green leafy vegetables (unwashed. Especially Dandelion)
- Ormus Greens
- Vitamineral Green

Excellent Sources of Protein (Amino Acids)

- Spirulina
- Bee pollen
- Goji Berries
- Maca
- Hemp seeds
- Quinoa
- Almonds
- Pumpkin seeds
- Chlorella
- Blue-Green Algae
- Sun Warrior Protein
- Hemp Protein
- Sprouts (all types)
- Aloe vera
- Ormus Greens

Freedom to Succeed

This is an incredibly empowering time because you have the opportunity to create the body, the health, and the life that you truly want to have. To put it simply, what you are eating is *fueling your ultimate path,* and it's going to determine the expression of your physical body, as well as the type of life that you will be participating in from here on out. When you honor your body with the best nutrition, then getting in shape becomes unexplainably simple. With the combination of exercise, a positive vision of yourself (and appreciation for your body and the health that you already have), plus so much incredible food to eat with nothing but health benefits…You can only succeed! You have to understand that you already have all of the potential within you. You truly know what's right for your body, mind, and consciousness. Give your body what it deserves, and you will receive benefits far beyond what you can imagine!

Enjoy the Best Food in the World! You know what it is now. If you don't know everything (which no one ever does), then set out on your own passionate exploration. Take some time out to find out about *you.* Become an expert on yourself. Find out how to uncover the truth within *you;* that you are healthy, happy, and already complete. It's an incredible journey; filled with truth, fulfillment, insight, and transformation. What you have already done by reading this book is set in motion the manifestation of situations and circumstances that will enable you to transcend the story of "all of my past struggles," so that you can get away from all of the illusions that have labeled you as less-than for far too long. This book is an instrument of manifestation.

Understand this with full clarity and comprehension for yourself and your family: **You Are What You Eat.** Lifeless, denatured foods simply do not have the energetic quality to create an environment of radiant health within you. When you eat that way, your body is more like a cemetery, not a place of vibrant life and vitality. The optimal foods for all of us are living, high-energy foods that actually have the ability to create new life.

It's phenomenal what you can create now with live foods. Not only that, just the sheer amount of foods, and new dishes that you can create with these foods is absolutely mind-blowing, and incredibly exciting once you become aware of them. Living on live food is not a gimmick, it's not just a fad diet that will get you some results and then taper off; or leave you sick, tired, and in regression, right back and likely worse off than where you began. *This is the reality:* Living food is what our bodies are designed to have. You have to unplug yourself from all of the hearsay, from all of the misinformation, from all of the marketing that has been subconsciously telling you what you should be eating since before you can remember.

The time is now for you to take your power back. Not your doctor, not your nutritionist, not your personal trainer, not your friends and family. Though these people can be beneficial along the way, in the end it is you who has to take responsibility for *you*.

Victor Hugo said, *"Nothing is more powerful than an idea whose time has come."* The time has come for the realization of The Key to Quantum Health. A transformation into true health consciousness, getting reconnected to what is real and sacred about each and every one of us, and living a life that is truly worthy of our infinite nature.

Make it a passion to seek out the most life-giving foods in the world. Find out how to bring them into your life, and enable these truths to manifest through *you*—incredible health, beauty, youth, vitality, and absolute abundance.

Enjoy Your Incredible Health, Love Life, and Appreciate all the things that you experience, and you will receive everything that you intend!

References

Enzyme Nutrition by Dr. Edward Howell
(Avery 1985)

Acid and Alkaline by Herman Aihara
(George Ohsawa Macrobiotic Foundation 1986)

Conscious Eating by Dr. Gabriel Cousens
(North Atlantic Books and Essene Vision Books 2000)

Survival into the 21st Century by Viktoras Kulvinskas
(21st Century Publication 2002)

Rainbow Green Live-Food Cuisine by Dr. Gabriel Cousens
(North Atlantic Books and Essene Vision Books 2003)

Eating for Beauty by David Wolfe
(Sunfood Publishing 2007)

Water: The Foundation of Youth, Health, and Beauty
by William D. Holloway, Jr. & Herb Joiner-Bey, ND
(IMPAKT Health 2004)

Vibrant Health by Dr. Norman Walker
(Norwalk Press 1995)

LifeFood Recipe Book by Annie Padding Jubb and David Jubb
(North Atlantic Books 2003)

The Sunfood Diet Success System by David Wolfe
(Maul Brothers Publishing 2006)

Proverbs 23:7 (English Revised Version)

The Life Visioning Process by Michael Beckwith
(Sounds True and Agape Media International 2008)

Organically Grown Food: It really is better for you! (Gerson Research Organization 1989)

DietFailureTheNakedTruth.com (Phoenix Gilman)

Enzyme Power for Digestion and Nutrient Absorption (Elisabeth Hsu-LeBlanc)

Encarta World Dictionary (English Version)

MSG: Slowly Poisoning America (rense.com)

The Water Cure (Interview with Dr. Batmanghelidj and Anthony Robbins)

Recommended Books (Health/Nutrition)

Stop Your Indigestion by Phyllis Avery

The Amazing Liver and Gallbladder Flush by Andreas Moritz

The Biology of Belief by Dr. Bruce Lipton

Recommended Books (Success/Right Thinking)

Think and Grow Rich by Napoleon Hill

Awaken the Giant Within by Anthony Robbins

Recommended Books (Spirituality/Meditation)

The Essene Gospel of Peace translation by Edmond Bordeaux Szekely

Inspiration: Your Ultimate Calling by Wayne Dyer

References

Being in Balance by Wayne Dyer

Life Visioning Process (Audio Recording) by Dr. Michael Beckwith

The Yoga of Jesus by Paramahansa Yogananda

A New Earth by Eckhart Tolle

For more information on meditation, research teachers like Michael Beckwith (www.agapelive.com), Thich Nhat Hanh, Wayne Dyer, Ram Das, and Deepak Chopra.

This is the greatest time ever to be alive because you can research any of these great teachers instantaneously. Simply go to youtube.com and check out some of their videos. When you find a teacher that resonates with you, support them, practice, and become the true embodiment of the potential that is within yourself.

Recommended Books (Recipes)

Rawvolution by Matt Amsden

Everyday Raw by Matthew Kinney

Living on Live Food by Alissa Cohen

Rainbow Green Live-Food Cuisine by Dr. Gabriel Cousens

Raw: The Uncook Book by Juliano

Additional Films I Highly Recommend

Healing Cancer from Inside Out Produced by Mike Anderson

The Future of Food Produced by Deborah Koons Garcia

Raw for Life visit simplyrawmovie.com

Simply Raw visit simplyrawmovie.com

Super Size Me Produced by Morgan Spurlock

Eating Produced by Mike Anderson

The Secret visit thesecret.tv

The Moses Code visit themosescode.com

What the Bleep Do We Know!? visit whatthebleep.com

Helpful Web Sites I Highly Recommend

www.TheShawnStevensonModel.com
www.naturalnews.com
www.thebestdayever.com
www.welikeitraw.com
www.goneraw.com
www.agapelilve.com
www.goveg.com
www.living-foods.com
www.ravediet.com
www.hippocratesinst.org
www.shiftinaction.com (Institute of Noetic Sciences)
www.treeoflife.nu

References

Many of the products mentioned are available online at www.TheShawnStevensonModel.com and at several of your local Health Food stores.

Highly recommended investments in your health and in making incredible food creations:
- Excalibur Dehydrator
- Cuisinart Food Processor
- Magic Bullet
- Jack LaLanne Power Juicer
- Vita-Mix Blender

About the Author

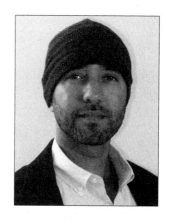

Shawn Stevenson is a Professional Nutritionist specializing in biochemistry and kinesiological science, as well as advanced treatment for acute and chronic disorders. He is the author of several books including *The Detox Success System* and *The Fat Loss Code*. He holds a Bachelors of Science degree from The University of Missouri – St. Louis, and he is the founder of the Advanced Integrative Health Alliance.

Over nearly a decade of research, Shawn's work has touched the lives of thousands of people in his private practice, programs, and live events. Shawn's greatest gift has been providing a tremendous array of valuable strategies, insights, techniques, tools for healing, and proven methods for radically transforming the health and beauty of the human body.

Shawn's mandate is that "If you're not growing, you're dying" and he is always passionately seeking and advocating the leading-edge sciences and wellness discoveries. His message and passion is communicated powerfully in his work, which has enabled Shawn to reach into institutions and communities to give solutions, hope, and empowerment at levels that have rarely been seen before.

Shawn recognizes that intelligent inspiration is not only valuable, but absolutely essential in our current environmental landscape to truly activate the potential of the great minds and leaders of the future.

To book Shawn Stevenson for radio, television, live seminars, or keynote speaking engagements please contact via email at: support@theshawnstevensonmodel.com

www.TheShawnStevensonModel.com

Over nearly a decade of research and working with thousands of people in my private practice and at live events, I've had the tremendous fortune of amassing a huge array of valuable strategies, insights, techniques, tools for healing, and methods for radically transforming the beauty of the human body.

The greatest gift that I could possibly give would be access to this information; to be able to help individuals turn years into days, and to radically transform the overall awareness on the planet. What I want to see is that what I have come to experience, and what my clients have come to enjoy, reveals itself as being the common experience in our culture. No longer is incredible health the exception, but it's the rule. And every man, woman, boy, and girl has the opportunity to truly be empowered and experience the greatest health and happiness possible.

This does not come from the old moniker "Knowledge is Power", this is realized through the real life application and experience of the knowledge... This comes from individuals being inspired enough to take action on what they want, and step-by-step coming to realize the genius within themselves. What this actually reveals is that "Knowledge ACTIVATED is Power". This is why I created this exclusive membership site that is available at www.TheShawnStevensonModel.com for membership registration.

All in one site you will have access to the absolute leading-edge information in health and longevity. You will have access to priceless information in the fields of nutrition, exercise technology, weight loss, peak performance, treatment of chronic and acute conditions, and much, much more.

Some of the information available to you here will give you the inside track on:

- Permanent weight loss and body fat reduction
- Detoxification and cleansing
- Advanced Anti-aging research
- Sexual health
- Optimal skin health (beauty and aesthetics)
- Leading-edge exercise instruction
- Major advancements in enhancing physical and mental energy
- Elite and rarely known diet information (discovering the system that works for YOU)
- Mental health (Improving mental clarity, awareness, and focus)

I know for certain that the greatest way to affect change in your life is through IMMERSION. To discover what it is that you want, and then to proactively put yourself in contact with that life as much as possible. This brings unimaginable speed to the realization of your dreams. The greatest investment is the investment in the health of yourself and your family. There is NOTHING more essential and honorable than that. If you are an individual who is interested in experiencing the most incredible health, connection, and happiness possible, become an exclusive part of the membership site to stay on the leading-edge of health and success. I'll see you inside!!!

Index

A

Acai, 124

Acid, 68, 93, 94, 96, 120, 128, 234

Adaptogen, 124

Adrenal, 25, 120

Allergies, 213

Alkaline, 151, 203, 215, 218, 234

Almond milk, 147, 150–152, 160, 177, 179, 180

Aloe Vera, 126, 155, 228, 231

Aliesthetic, 115, 214

Amino Acid, 68, 94–96, 117, 120–125, 128, 163, 231

— *Excellent Sources of,* 231

Anandamide, 120

Antioxidant, 120, 121, 123, 124, 126, 161

Aphrodisiac, 124

Apple Cider Vinegar, 125, 164, 165, 182, 184, 206, 208, 209, 212

Asthma, 32, 202, 213

B

Bacteria, 111, 124, 201

Barley, 149, 152, 188

Bee Pollen, 96, 121, 149, 152, 195, 231

Beta Carotene, 117, 121

Beta-Glucans, 152

Beauty Food, 109, 111, 113, 116, 227

Bioelectricity, 24

Biophoton, 27, 28, 31

Blue Mangosteen, 156

Blue-Green Algae, 129, 207, 209, 210, 231

Buddha, 101

C

Cacao, 118–121, 145, 148, 151, 153–159, 166, 193–195, 227–229

Camu Camu berries, 124, 201, 202, 205, 207–212, 217, 219–224, 229

Cancer, 17, 32, 88, 96, 97, 99, 105, 121, 122, 124, 158, 237

Candida, 158, 201

Cat's Claw, 158, 161, 162

Calcium, 91, 96, 97, 100, 114, 229

— *Foods rich in,* 229

Celtic Sea Salt, 127, 148, 160, 166, 168, 175, 176, 178, 181, 182, 184, 196, 205, 207–212, 217, 219–224

Clement, Dr. Brian, 17, 18

Chocolate, 118–121, 148–151, 153–158, 161, 162, 195, 207, 211, 220, 222

Cholesterol, 96, 97, 99, 122, 124

Cousens, Dr. Gabriel, 17, 18, 234, 236

Coconut, 123, 143–145, 148–150, 154, 157, 159, 165, 193, 227, 230

Coconut Oil, 116, 124, 148, 150, 152, 156, 158, 166, 230

Coconut water, 123, 145, 148, 150, 153, 154, 156, 157, 176, 195

Cordyceps, 129, 154, 155, 158

D

Dehydrator, 142, 238

Detoxification, 104, 147, 199, 212, 241

Detoxify, 126, 199

Diabetes, 17, 32, 97, 99, 100

Diet, 11, 12, 14, 21, 29, 34, 57, 58, 79, 97, 116, 125, 233–235, 237, 241

   – *Percent of Diets that Fail,* 57
   – *Standard American Diet (SAD), 21, 89, 93, 143,*

DNA, 28

Dyer, Dr. Wayne, 15, 50, 235, 236

E

Edestin, 122

Energy Source, 115, 116, 214

Enzyme, 29–32, 83–85, 90, 96, 106, 113–116, 123, 163, 167, 172, 180, 188, 206, 208–211, 215, 219–221, 223, 224, 226, 234, 235

Enzyme Inhibitors, 188

80/20 Raw Options, 186

Einstein, Albert, 65, 97

Essential Fatty Acids (EFA's), 114, 116, 230

   – *Excellent Sources of,* 230

Excitotoxins, 100

Exercise, 11, 12, 45, 72, 129, 199, 200, 216, 218, 226, 232, 240, 241

F

Fiber, 93, 124, 137, 166, 172, 225

Flying High Smoothie, 149, 221, 223

Free Radicals, 96, 99, 126

Fungus, 124, 201

Index

G
Garlic, 124, 164, 167, 171, 174, 175, 177–186, 228, 229

Genetically Modified Organisms (GMO's), 88, 90

Goji Berries, 117, 118, 123, 144, 145, 147, 149–152, 155, 159, 161, 193–196, 220, 221, 223, 229–231

H
Hemp seeds, 122, 145, 148, 149, 154, 155, 158, 159, 178, 183, 194, 217, 220, 222, 228, 230, 231

High Fructose Corn Syrup, 99, 214

Honey, 120, 123, 145, 148, 155–159, 167, 177, 180–182, 184, 185, 194, 195, 230

Human Growth Hormone (HGH), 118, 199, 225

I
Immune System, 26, 32, 125, 126, 152, 163, 201

Iodine, 125

Inca, 124, 144, 145, 196, 220, 221, 223

Iron, 91, 111, 227
 – *Foods rich in,* 227

J
Juice Recipes, 189

K
Kelp, 125, 164–166, 169, 173, 174, 178, 183, 212, 219, 220, 228

Kirlian Field Photography, 24, 26, 66

Kulvinskas, Viktoras, 14, 18, 234

Kombucha, 126, 230

L
Lean Muscle, 200

Living Food, 17–19, 21, 28, 30, 32, 84, 115, 233, 237

Longevity, 105, 107, 123, 126, 129, 155, 199, 202, 208, 209, 217, 240

M
Maca, 124, 145, 148, 150, 151, 153–159, 195, 205, 228, 231

Magnesium, 91, 119, 229
 – *Best Sources of,* 229

Mangosteen, 126, 156

Manganese, 111, 228
 – *Foods rich in,* 228

Meditation, 3, 78, 136, 137, 212, 235, 236

Metabolic, 83, 122, 125, 200

Methylsulfonylmethane (MSM), 201, 202, 205, 207–212, 217, 219–224

MSG, 99, 100, 235

Muscle Mass, 225
 – Menu For Increasing, 217, 219–224
 – Additional Tips For Building, 225

N

Neurotransmitter, 120

Neuro-Tissue, 114

Noni, 123

O

Omega-3 and 6 *(also see Essential Fatty Acids)*, 116, 112, 124

Quinoa, 124, 157, 231

Ormus Greens, 150, 151, 153–156, 159, 190, 191, 230, 231

Organic Food, 88–90, 192, 196
 – *Importance of,* 87

P

Partially Hydrogenated Oil, 99

Pasteurized Dairy Products, 93, 96, 213

Phenylethylamine (PEA), 120

Photodegrade, 105

Phytochemcials, 24, 96

Polysaccharides, 123, 126

Popp, Fritz-Albert, 28

Protein *(also see Amino Acid)*, 83, 84, 91, 94–96, 100, 106, 117, 121, 122, 124, 127, 128, 144, 147–153, 163, 213, 217, 219, 224, 231

Processed Sugar, 25, 115, 215

Prebiotics, 230

Plant Foods/Animal Foods comparison, 96

Probiotics, 126, 201, 215, 225, 230
 – *Excellent Sources of,* 230

Q

Quantum Physics, 1, 41, 65, 67, 135

R

Raw Foods *(also see Living Foods)* 83, 142, 143, 146, 214

S

SAD Diet, 21, 89, 93, 143

Salad Dressings, 121–124

Schuphan, Werner, 90

Sea Salt *(also see Celtic Sea Salt)*, 127, 149, 151–155, 157, 166, 167, 170–172, 174, 177, 178, 180, 182, 183, 194, 195

Index

Sea Vegetables, 125, 143, 227–229

Serotonin, 120

Silicon, 111, 228
– Foods rich in, 228

Skin (Health), 106, 241

Smoothies (also see Superfood Smoothies), 118, 120–124, 148–151, 195, 197, 203, 221, 223

Spirulina, 96, 121, 190, 227, 228, 231

Sulfur, 111, 183, 201, 202, 228
– Foods rich in, 228

Sun Warrior Protein, 127, 128, 147–153, 163, 231

Superfood Shakes/Smoothies, 123, 195, 197, 203

Superfoods, 4, 26, 117
– Desciption of, 117
– Benefits of, 117

T

The Detox Success System, 199, 216, 239

The Shawn Stevenson Model, 212, 123, 129, 137, 200, 203, 215, 216, 226, 237–240

Thyroid, 124, 125

UV

Vitamin C, 91, 119, 202, 229
– Foods rich in, 229

Vitamineral Green, 190, 230

Vegetarian, 97

Vita-Mix, 142, 238

W

Water
– Benefits of, 103

Wheat Grass, 227

Weight Gain, 91

Weight Loss, 107, 120, 126, 240, 241
– Menus For, 205, 207–212
– Additional Tips For, 213

Wigmore, Ann, 18, 143

X

Xenoestrogens, 105

Y

Yacon, 150, 151, 153, 154, 230

Z

Zinc, 111, 112, 227
– Foods rich in, 227